Oxford Medical Engineering Series

EDITORS: B. McA. Sayers
P. Cliffe

The study of heart-rate variability

EDITED BY
R. I. KITNEY
AND

O. ROMPELMAN

CLARENDON PRESS · OXFORD
1980

LQL K

Oxford University Press, Walton Street, Oxford OX2 6DP
OXFORD LONDON GLASGOW
NEW YORK TORONTO MELBOURNE WELLINGTON
KUALA LUMPUR SINGAPORE JAKARTA HONG KONG TOKYO
DELHI BOMBAY CALCUTTA MADRAS KARACHI
IBADAN NAIROBI DAR ES SALAAM CAPE TOWN

Published in the United States by Oxford University Press, New York.

British Library Cataloguing in Publication Data
The study of heart-rate variability. – (Oxford
  medical engineering series).
  1. Arrhythmia
  I. Kitney, R I   II. Rompelman, O
  616.1'28   RC685.A65   80–40261

ISBN 0–19–857533–5

Filmset by Universities Press, Belfast
Printed in Great Britain by
Lowe & Brydone Printers Ltd, Thetford, Norfolk

Preface

THE nature and origin of fluctuations in heart-rate, or as it is now known, heart-rate variability (HRV), have become increasingly of interest in recent years. Heart-rate variability is now often considered as one of the number of physiological parameters that mirror the response of the human cardiovascular system to more-or-less definable stimuli, these stimuli being physical, psychological, or environmental. The spontaneous fluctuations that occur in heart-rate have been studied extensively and from this work it has become clear that several factors other than simply respiration affect heart-rate. Correspondingly, the effects of stimuli and their interactions with components of the spontaneous activity offer possibilities for insight into biological mechanisms and the prospect of useful application.

In 1977 the Biological Engineering Society held a meeting at Chelsea College, London, on the analysis of heart-rate variability. This was attended by workers from a wide range of disciplines: physiology, psychology, psychiatry, clinical medicine, engineering, and physics. The meeting revealed a wide-ranging interest in HRV; most of the chapters in the book are based upon papers presented at the meeting and the rest were invited to provide a more comprehensive survey of the subject. The objective of the book is to consider the physiological and engineering backgrounds of the field, as well as to show some examples of applications. Since in different chapters HRV is examined from different points of view, it is inevitable not only that overlap will occur but also that some contradictions will emerge. But the general aim of the book is to present some important aspects of the state of the art, rather than to provide, in any sense, a complete textbook on the subject.

The text is divided into four parts: background physiology, analysis techniques, applications with respect to physiology, and other applications. The first part begins with a contribution from Dr Alastair McDonald (Senior Lecturer in Cardiology, The London Hospital). In this chapter the mechanisms affecting heart-rate are considered under three general headings: intrinsic cardiac mechanisms, cardiovascular reflexes, and integrated cardiovascular responses. Following on this discussion of cardiovascular control at the macroscopic level, the next chapter deals with a more microscopic matter—the generation of the action potential at the sino-atrial node. Dr Noble (Oxford University), the author of the chapter, is doubly qualified for this task because, in addition to his published textbook, *The initiation of the heartbeat*, his researches have made him a leading international authority on this aspect of physiology. Starting with the work of Gaskell in 1883, the rhythmic firing of the sino-atrial node is discussed in terms of a slow depolarization following each action potential. The ionic mechanism of the pacemaker potential has been the subject of intensive research since the application of the voltage-clamp technique to cardiac muscle in 1964. In this chapter Noble examines how different transmitters such as adrenaline, noradrenaline, and acetylcholine achieve control of heart-rate at the ionic level, and also the role of cardiac glycosides in this context.

The second part of the book covers the analysis techniques which are used in the study of heart-rate variability. To this end, Professor Sayers (Imperial College) was asked to provide a survey chapter on this topic. In his paper, Sayers considers the nature of the heart-rate signal, through the analysis of both its long-term and its short-term properties.

The theme of analysis techniques continues with the contribution of Ir Rompelman (Delft). In his chapter two main topics are considered: the best way to extract the interval information from the ECG, and the most appropriate methods of analysis for a particular derived HRV signal. A method for the extraction of HRV is introduced which is based on a particular model of the SA node. The basis of model is that heart-rate is primarily altered by autonomic activity. The concept of spontaneously oscillating physiological control systems which are believed to be largely responsible for HRV is also discussed, and analysis techniques which are specifically designed to cope with non-stationary oscillations, e.g. complex demodulation and homomorphic filtering are introduced.

The third part of the book considers the role of heart-rate variability within the wider context of the regulation of arterial blood pressure. The first section of the chapter by Dr Kitney (Imperial College, London) deals with the thermoregulatory influence on heart-rate which has been found to lie in the frequency range 0–0·1 Hz. Kitney discusses the oscillatory behaviour which occurs in the thermoregulatory system: this is thought to emanate from a non-linear control system which is responsible to external influences. The second aspect of his contribution is on analysis of the oscillatory behaviour of physiological control systems. The control theory model introduced in Chapter 4, which describes the nature of the physiological oscillations, is presented and its development discussed from both the physiological and control points of view. The final section of this chapter comprises a discussion of the relationship between metastable and unstable entrainment in the light of this control theory model.

The chapter by Professor P. Sleight (Oxford), discusses the physiology of heart-rate control in man and animals by arterial baroreceptors. Sleight also describes how when blood-pressure is perturbed during steady-state conditions there is a linear relationship between systolic blood-pressure and pulse interval. The slope of this relation can be used as a quantitative measure of the gain of the reflex arc. Gain is found to be greatest during sleep, particularly during dreams, and is diminished by upright posture. It is also greatly reduced by exercise and mental activity. The effect of certain drugs on the gain of the baroreflex arc is described. For example, the therapeutic action of clonidine seems to lie in increasing the gain. Sleight also discusses stiffness in the arterial wall as a possible cause of hypertension because it is the site of the sensory receptors.

The final part of the book covers other aspects of heart-rate variability analysis. The first chapter in this section is by Dr G. H. Byford of the Royal Air Force Institute of Aviation Medicine. In it he describes the pitfalls that can occur in HRV analysis. These include variations in R-wave timing due to changes in ECG shape and deviations from normality when considering a series of RR intervals. The relative value of the analysis of HRV when placed in the right perspective is discussed, which makes this contribution a valuable one.

In Chapter 8 Professor Luczak, Dr Philipp, and Professor Rohmert (Darmstadt) consider the decomposition of heart-rate variability under ergonomic aspects of stressor analysis. First ergonomic aspects of HRV are dealt with and this is followed by the introduction of a model which describes the interaction of the cardiovascular and respiratory systems. The second half of the chapter covers a number of experimental and analytical methods which are designed to score HRV and divide the phenomenon into various constituent parts.

The chapter by Dr A. Roscoe of the Royal Aircraft Establishment, Bedford, describes work which has been carried out on test pilots over the last 8 years. In this research the heart-rates of test pilots were monitored while flying experimental sorties. The results, together with subjective ratings by the pilots, have been used to estimate and compare levels of workload.

Dr B. W. Hyndman of the TNO, Leiden, discusses in Chapter 10 the assessment of mental load by means of spectral analysis of HRV records. The author describes the effect of a 3-minute cognitive task on the spectral content of successive R waves of the ECG in healthy human subjects. The results of these experiments showed significant changes in the 7–10-s band. These changes lasted for about 45 minutes after the task performance period. The physiological meaning and its implications for hypertension research are also discussed.

The final chapter is by Dr R. Offerhaus, who is a psychiatrist with long experience on HRV applications in psychiatry. Offerhaus considers the problem of distinguishing the mentally ill from the healthy and how HRV analysis can be used to this end. Specifically he considers the analysis of HRV data obtained in an experimental situation employing mental load (binary choice task), followed by a period of rest, for this purpose. A statistical analysis of heart-rate data evidently confirms the applicability of HRV analysis in this field.

The book finishes with some concluding remarks by the editors.

London   R.I.K.
Delft   O.R.
April 1979

Contents

LIST OF CONTRIBUTORS   xiii

PART I
BACKGROUND PHYSIOLOGY

1. MECHANISMS AFFECTING HEART-RATE   3
A. H. McDONALD
1.1. Introduction. 1.2. Intrinsic mechanisms. 1.3. Cardiovascular reflexes.
1.4. Integrated responses. 1.5. Conclusion.

2. BIOPHYSICAL MECHANISMS CONTROLLING
HEART-RATE AND ITS VARIABILITY   13
D. NOBLE
2.1. Introduction. 2.2. Ionic channels involved in pacemaker activity.
2.3. Autonomic transmitters. 2.4 Cardiac glycosides. 2.5 Conclusion.

PART II
TECHNIQUES OF ANALYSIS

3. SIGNAL ANALYSIS OF HEART-RATE VARIABILITY   27
B. McA. SAYERS
3.1. The nature of the heart-rate signal. 3.2. Statistical techniques of
analysis. 3.3. Signal measures. 3.4. Pattern analysis. 3.5. Conclusion.

4. THE ASSESSMENT OF FLUCTUATIONS IN
HEART-RATE   59
O. ROMPELMAN
4.1. Introduction. 4.2. HRV signals. 4.3. The integral pulse frequency
modulator model (IPFM). 4.4. The concept of spontaneous oscillating control systems applied to heart-rate variability. 4.5. Signal analysis
methods. 4.6. Conclusion.

PART III
APPLICATIONS OF HEART-RATE VARIABILITY ANALYSIS
WITH RESPECT TO PHYSIOLOGY

5. AN ANALYSIS OF THE THERMOREGULATORY
INFLUENCES ON HEART-RATE VARIABILITY   81
R. I. KITNEY
5.1. Introduction. 5.2. Analysis of the three types of entrainment. 5.3. The
control theory basis of the mechanism. 5.4. Analysis of the model by

CONTENTS

describing function techniques. 5.5. The relationship between metastable and unstable entrainment. 5.6. Conclusion.

6. THE PHYSIOLOGY OF HEART-RATE CONTROL BY ARTERIAL BARORECEPTORS IN MAN AND ANIMALS   107
P. SLEIGHT
6.1. Introduction. 6.2. Historical review. 6.3. Receptor Physiology. 6.4. Conclusion.

PART IV
OTHER ASPECTS OF HEART-RATE VARIABILITY ANALYSIS

7. HEART-RATE AND ITS VARIABILITY—PITFALLS, ETC.   117
G. H. BYFORD
7.1. Introduction. 7.2. Problems in using ECG measurements. 7.3. Problems in statistical analysis of heart-rate. 7.4. Conclusion.

8. DECOMPOSITION OF HEART-RATE VARIABILITY UNDER THE ERGONOMIC ASPECTS OF STRESSOR ANALYSIS   123
H. LUCZAK, U. PHILIPP, AND W. ROHMERT
8.1. Introduction: scales of heart-rate variation. 8.2. Research approach to heart-rate variation (HRV) in ergonomic terms. 8.3. Analysis of a model of the cardiovascular and cardiorespiratory system. 8.4. Experiments on superimposition of components of stress. 8.5. Polygraphic assessment of physiological indicators of arousal. 8.6. Conclusion.

9. HEART-RATE CHANGES IN TEST PILOTS   178
A. H. ROSCOE
9.1. Introduction 9.2. Heart-rate as a measure of pilot workload. 9.3. Sinus arrhythmia as a measure of pilot workload. 9.4. Conclusion.

10. CARDIOVASCULAR RECOVERY TO PSYCHOLOGICAL STRESS: A MEANS TO DIAGNOSE MAN AND TASK?   191
B. W. HYNDMAN
10.1. Introduction. 10.2. Signal-processing of the cardiac event sequence. 10.3. The blood-pressure fluctuations. 10.4. Cardiovascular disturbances of physiological origin. 10.5. Non-invasive blood-pressure measurement. 10.6. Analysis of the arterial blood-pressure signal.

11. HEART-RATE VARIABILITY IN PSYCHIATRY 225
R. E. OFFERHAUS
11.1. Introduction.   11.2. Methods and procedures.   11.3. Results.

CONCLUDING REMARKS 239

INDEX 241

List of contributors

G. H. BYFORD — RAF Institute of Aviation Medicine, Farnborough, Hampshire.

B. W. HYNDMAN — Netherlands Organization for Health Research, TNO, Leiden, The Netherlands.

R. I. KITNEY — Engineering in Medicine Laboratory, Imperial College, London.

H. LUCZAK — Institut für Arbeitswissenschaft, Technische Hochschule, Darmstadt, FRG. (Presently with the Forschungsstelle und Laboratorium für Produktionstechnik, Universität Bremen, FRG.)

A. H. McDONALD — Cardiac Department, The London Hospital, London.

D. NOBLE — University Laboratory of Physiology, Oxford University, Oxford.

R. E. OFFERHAUS — Psychiatric Centre, St. Bavo, Noordwijkerhout, The Netherlands. (Presently with the Municipal Department of Social Psychiatry, Rotterdam, The Netherlands.)

U. PHILIPP — Institut für Arbeitswissenschaft, Technische Hochschule, Darmstadt, FRG.

W. ROHMERT — Institut für Arbeitswissenschaft, Technische Hochschule, Darmstadt, FRG.

O. ROMPELMAN — Department of Electrical Engineering. Delft University of Technology, The Netherlands.

A. H. ROSCOE — Royal Aircraft Establishment, Bedford, Hampshire.

B. McA. SAYERS — Engineering in Medicine Laboratory, Imperial College, London.

P. SLEIGHT — Department of Cardiovascular Medicine, University of Oxford.

Part I

Background physiology

1.
Mechanisms affecting heart-rate
A. H. McDONALD

1.1. Introduction

THE purpose of this introductory chapter is to provide a brief summary of the chief mechanisms affecting the heart-rate. These mechanisms are complex and, while there are detailed studies of some systems in isolation, the integrated actions of different influences remains sketchily understood.

In crude terms the mechanisms influencing heart-rate can be divided into three categories: the intrinsic cardiac mechanisms which are the source of cardiac rhythmicity; the cardiovascular reflexes which are the basis of circulatory control and mediated principally by the medullary vasomotor centres; and integrated patterns of cardiovascular response to a variety of functional demands such as exercise or thermal regulation which involve higher neural centres.

Hormonal influences such as circulating catecholamines and thyroxine will also affect the heart-rate, either by direct action on the heart or indirectly by more general effects on metabolism.

1.2. Intrinsic mechanisms

In Chapter 2 of this volume the initiation of the heart-rate is dealt with in much greater detail. Automaticity is a fundamental property of the myocardium but is not present to an equal degree in all cells. For present purposes, dealing with normal heart-rate control, the sino-atrial node (Fig. 1.1) lying at the junction of the superior vena cava and the right atrium is the pacemaker, the driving force of the heart's rhythm. Other cardiac cells exhibit automaticity—for example, atrial cells along the internodal tracts, junctional cells in the region of atrio-ventricular node, cells in the bundle of His, and ventricular Purkinje cells—but the sino-atrial node normally has the highest spontaneous discharge rate.

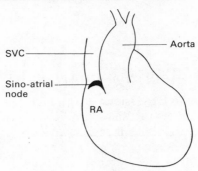

FIG. 1.1. Diagram of the heart to show the position of the sino-atrial node at the junction of the superior vena cava (SVC) and the right atrium (RA).

The basis of automaticity in the sino-atrial node is spontaneous depolarization of the cell membrane during diastole. Fig. 1.2 is a schematic representation of intracellular recordings of the membrane potential in cardiac cells. The non-pacemaker cell has a more negative resting potential, about $-100\,\text{mV}$, a rapid rate of depolarization, and a prolonged recovery or repolarization. The non-pacemaker will produce an action potential only when it is depolarized by the arrival of the wave of excitation from neighbouring cells. In contrast the pacemaker cell has a resting potential nearer to the threshold potential for the initiation of an action potential. The main attribute of the pacemaker cell is the slow spontaneous diastolic depolarization. The discharge rate and therefore the heart-rate depends on the slope of diastolic depolarization.

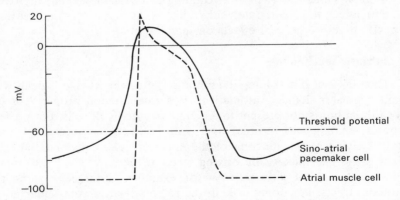

FIG. 1.2 Schematic representation of the membrane potential of a sino-atrial muscle cell (pacemaker cell) and atrial muscle cell (non-pacemaker cell).

Structurally the sino-atrial node is composed of dense fibrous tissue in which small interweaving muscle fibres are embedded. A functional curiosity is the close relationship of the sino-atrial nodal artery which is aligned to the node passing roughly through the long axis. This may simply reflect a primitive origin as a neurovascular bundle but it is a large vessel in relation to the dimensions of the node. It has been suggested that external pulsation in the sino-atrial nodal artery can entrain the discharge rate of the node, but it seems unlikely that this occurs within the physiological direct pressure range. This possible mechanical feedback to the node has not been given detailed study.

The spontaneous heart-rate shows marked species difference but in general terms is inversely related to mass. This is also true of man, infants having a higher resting heart-rate than children, and children having faster rates than adults. The maximum heart-rate which can be achieved by maximal exercise shows a progressive fall with age (Fig. 1.3). At age

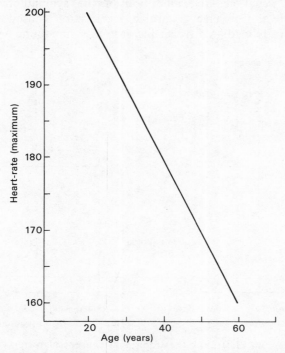

FIG. 1.3. The effect of age on the maximum heart-rate achieved by maximal exercise.

20 years the maximum heart-rate will be about 200 beats per minute but falls by about 10 beats per decade so that, at age 60 years, the maximum is only 160 beats per minute. There is, however, a wide range for any age group which makes it impossible to predict the maximum heart-rate for a given individual.

The rate of discharge of the sino-atrial node is controlled by the dual innervation from the vagus nerve, which is inhibitory and slows the heart, and the sympathetic, which is excitatory and increases the rate. Traditionally, (Fig. 1.4) the relationship between the two neural influences was considered to be a simple reciprocal variation in the tonic effects of the vagus and sympathetic. In a series of experiments (Glick and Braunwald 1965) using autonomic blockade in anaesthetized and unanaesthetized animals as well as in human subjects, the reciprocal arrangement was disputed and an alternative relationship proposed (Fig. 1.4). This implies that cardiac slowing, induced by an acute rise in arterial pressure, is due to increased vagal activity, inhibition of the sympathetic having no important effect. Conversely, cardiac acceleration caused by a fall in blood-pressure is mediated by an increase in sympathetic activity rather

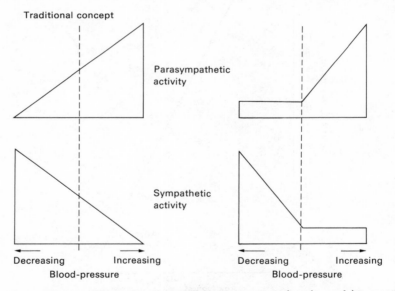

FIG. 1.4. Diagram illustrating the traditional concept of reciprocal innervation of the heart as compared to that based on studies of autonomic blockade (*right*). (Redrawn from Glick and Braunwald (1965).)

than by vagal withdrawal. Whether this relationship is correct, or there is an exponential or two involved, is not critical but it is the balance between the level of vagal and sympathetic activity which determines the heart-rate. The responses of the heart-rate control systems will be greatly affected by the relative dominance of either the vagus or the sympathetic. This will be markedly influenced by experimental conditions such as anaesthesia, drugs, and surgery. As a result much animal work may not give a suitable experimental model to study this interrelationship.

1.3. Cardiovascular reflexes

Numerous reflexes affecting the circulation have been described but demonstration does not mean that they have any significant part to play in man. There are recent critical reviews of the reflex control of the circulation (Abboud, Heistad, Mark, and Schmid 1976; Linden 1976). Afferent impulses arise from a number of receptor sites (Table 1.1) and their central connection is principally with medullary cardiovascular centres. The total effect of the afferent activity depends not only on the activity of peripheral receptors but also on inputs from higher centres. As a result of complex interaction among the afferent traffic, some synergistic, some inhibitory, and certainly not a simple algebraic summation, efferent activity arises. Again the effect is not a stereotype. Two excitatory outputs, while qualitatively similar, may produce effects which are different quantitatively; for example differential vasoconstriction in different regional circulations, or sympathetic stimulation which produces a tachycardia without peripheral vasoconstriction.

While the efferent neural control of the heart-rate has been appreciated for over 100 years it was only with Hering's discovery of the carotid sinus

TABLE 1.1
Some cardiovascular reflexes

Reflex	Receptor site
Baroreceptor reflex	Carotid sinus Aorta
Chemoreceptor reflex	Carotid body
Cardiac reflexes	(a) Atria (b) Ventricles
Respiratory sinus arrhythmia	? Lungs ? Atria

nerves in 1923 that the afferent side of the tonically active baroreceptor reflex began to be elucidated. The baroreceptor reflex has been studied in great detail. Essentially, it can be described as a buffer, protecting the body, and especially the brain, from excessive swings in the systemic arterial pressure. A rise in pressure causes bradycardia and promotes a drop in pressure by a reduction in peripheral vasoconstriction. The force of cardiac contraction is reduced by withdrawal of the positive inotropic effects of the sympathetic. A fall in arterial pressure produces opposite effects.

The chemoreceptors in the carotid body are stimulated by hypoxia, hypercapnia, and acidosis. The circulatory effects are excitatory but the chemoreceptors are principally involved with respiratory control. Within normal conditions they have minimal cardiovascular effects though it has been proposed that during severe exercise the reflex may provide an additional excitatory boost.

The reflexes arising from cardiac receptors continue to cause much dispute and their role in the control of the circulation is uncertain in many respects. Bainbridge in 1915 claimed to demonstrate reflex tachycardia from atrial distension caused by rapid infusion of saline, but the general circulatory effects of the infusion made interpretation difficult. Further studies failed to confirm this reflex adequately but recently careful and extensive studies (Linden 1976) have firmly established the reflex experimentally. Atrial mechanoreceptors at the junction of the vena cava and right atrium, and around the pulmonary veno-atrial junctions, when stimulated by distension of small balloons, produce a tachycardia. The afferent pathway is via the vagus and the cardiac acceleration is mediated by sympathetic stimulation. The same atrial receptors are the source of the reflex diuresis and it is believed that their major role is in blood volume regulation.

The ventricular cardiac receptors are anatomically poorly differentiated and their normal functional role unknown. It is believed that they are mechanoreceptors and their stimulation by ischaemia is a secondary phenomenon. They produce a depressor reflex (Bezold–Jarisch reflex) resulting in bradycardia and hypotension. Clinical counterparts may be involved in patients following cardiac infarction and after the intracoronary injection of contrast material.

Respiratory sinus arrhythmia appears to be a simple oscillation in the heart-rate (Fig. 1.5) and it is a major component of heart-rate variability. The mechanism of the reflex has not been established although the efferent pathway is in the vagus, the cardiac acceleration with inspiration

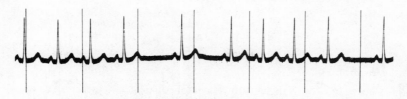

FIG. 1.5. Electrocardiogram, lead II showing variation in the heart-rate related to respiration.

being due to release of vagal tone and being totally blocked by atropinization. It has been suggested that it is a lung inflation reflex in that the afferent pathway is from pulmonary or respiratory tract receptors but positive pressure ventilation does not stimulate the reflex. Alternatively the variation in the heart-rate reflects respiratory modulation of the baroreceptor reflex. It has recently been proposed (Melcher 1976) that changes in intrathoracic pressure which induces changes in cardiac filling is the main stimulus to the reflex from stimulation of atrial receptors. Respiratory sinus arrhythmia is an age-dependent phenomenon. In an older subject (Fig. 1.6(a)) with a high resting vagal tone there is little respiratory variation in heart-rate but in a younger subject, despite a higher resting heart-rate, there is quite marked variation (Fig. 1.6(b)).

1.4. Integrated responses

The integrated responses of the cardiovascular system are more complex mechanisms involving supra-medullary centres notably the hypothalamus. Examples of these integrated responses are muscular exercise and thermoregulation but would also include the response to emotion and digestion.

At the onset of exercise the heart-rate increases abruptly and thereafter rises progressively with the level of exercise, (Fig. 1.7). Apart from the onset of exercise and near maximal levels there is a virtual linear relationship between heart-rate and the work load. This association is true of physically fit and unfit subjects although the slope of the line differs. During exercise there is a remarkable adjustment between local autoregulatory mechanisms in the exercising muscle and the central control systems. This adaptation continues after the cessation of exercise so the cardiac output response is finely graded to metabolic demands.

The limiting factors to exercise capability are skeletal muscle metabolism, limited energy source, and the demands of thermoregulation. As

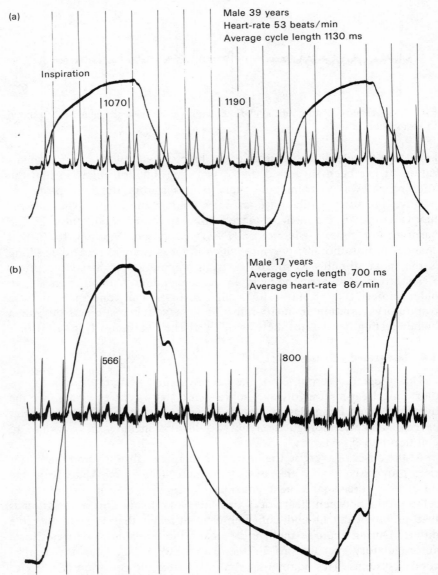

(a)

Male 39 years
Heart-rate 53 beats/min
Average cycle length 1130 ms

Inspiration

|1070| | 1190 |

(b)

Male 17 years
Average cycle length 700 ms
Average heart-rate 86/min

|566| |800|

FIG. 1.6. Electrocardiogram and respiratory trace. (a) Male aged 39 years showing slight variation only. (b) Male aged 17 years showing marked respiratory variation.

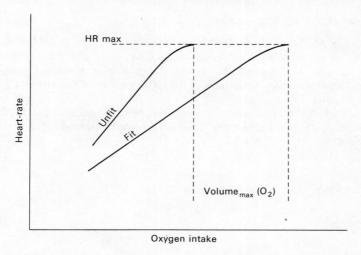

Fɪɢ. 1.7. Diagram showing the relation of increasing work load (oxygen intake) and heart rate in fit and unfit subjects.

heat production increases with higher levels of exercise the blood flow to the skin progressively increases so as to promote heat loss by radiation and evaporation of sweat. This means that proportionally less of the cardiac output is available for the exercising muscle and finally muscle blood flow will be inadequate to sustain further effort. Excluding diseased states cardiorespiratory factors are not limiting in the strict sense.

1.5. Conclusion

This chapter has outlined the main organizational levels of the control mechanisms affecting the heart-rate. It is clear that while our understanding of some areas is considerable there are many shadowy areas. Classical physiological analysis isolates the response under study, proves its existence, and defines the potential range of activity. However the experimental conditions of much animal work is likely to distort our understanding of the integrated function of the circulation. There is as yet little information about the relative dominance or priority when cardiovascular responses and reflexes interact. Inevitably this can be studied only in an intact preparation. The methods of analysis which are the subject of this volume may enable us to analyse the mechanisms affecting the heart-rate in the human subject in a more detailed manner.

References

ABBOUD, F. M., HEISTAD, D. D., MARK, A. L., and SCHMID, P. G. (1976). Reflex control of the peripheral circulation. *Prog. Cardiovasc. Dis.* **18,** 371–403.

GLICK, G. and BRAUNWALD, E. (1965). Relative roles of the sympathetic and para sympathetic nervous systems in the reflex control of heart-rate. *Circulation Res.* **16,** 363–75.

LINDEN, R. J. (1976). Reflexes from the heart. *Prog. Cardiovasc. Dis.* **18,** 201–21.

MELCHER, A. (1976). Respiratory sinus arrhythmia in man. *Acta Physiol. Scand. Suppl.* **435.**

2.
Biophysical mechanisms controlling heart-rate and its variability
D. NOBLE

2.1. Introduction

IT is now widely accepted that the mechanism of rhythmic activity in the heart lies in the muscular tissue of the sino-atrial node rather than in the activity of intracardiac ganglia and nerves. We owe this knowledge originally to W. H. Gaskell who reached this conclusion in 1883 following a series of experiments on frogs and tortoises. The role of the nervous system is rather to modulate the frequency of the inherent rhythmic activity. Interestingly enough, it was also W. H. Gaskell (1887) who first demonstrated a biophysical basis for this control since he was the first to demonstrate the hyperpolarizing action of the vagus nerve (for a recent account of this work see Banister, Brown, Giles, Hutter, and S. J. Noble 1976).

The immediate cause of rhythmic firing is known to be the development of a slow depolarization following each action potential. This depolarization is called the pacemaker potential. Each time the depolarization reaches the threshold for excitation a new action potential arises and the cycle recommences. The ionic mechanism of the pacemaker potential has been the subject of intensive study since the introduction of the voltage clamp technique in cardiac muscle in 1964 (Deck and Trautwein 1964). I have recently discussed some of this work in my book *The initiation of the heartbeat* (Noble 1979) and I shall not therefore give an extensive account here. Instead, I shall briefly draw attention to those features of the ionic mechanisms that may be relevant to a discussion of heart-rate variability.

2.2. Ionic channels involved in pacemaker activity

Although there are important quantitative differences, experiments on the different regions of the heart that show pacemaker activity all agree on one major fact. During each action potential a potassium conductance is activated that decays slowly during the pacemaker potential itself. This is illustrated in Fig. 2.1 which shows the result of an experiment in which pacemaker activity is interrupted by holding the membrane voltage constant at the end of the action potential. It is evident that this procedure is accompanied by the decay of an outward current. The negative reversal potential of this current strongly suggests that it is a potassium current.

By itself, an outward potassium current hyperpolarizes the membrane. Its decay can only lead to the development of a slow depolarization if it unmasks the presence of an inward ionic current. The origin of the inward current involved in pacemaker activity is still not entirely clear, but it appears necessary to distinguish between three different inward current mechanisms that may be involved.

(a) Some inward current in cardiac muscle flows more or less continuously and is not time-dependent. This current is usually called the inward

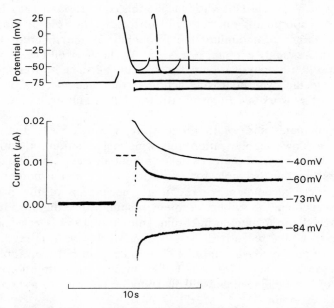

FIG. 2.1. Voltage clamp analysis of pacemaker current in frog atrium. The clamp was applied at various potentials at the end of the first action potential in each train. Outward current is shown as an upward deflection. Potentials positive with respect to −73 mV produce a decaying outward current that is thought to be carried by potassium ions. (Brown, Clark, and S. J. Noble 1972.)

background current (see Noble 1979, Chapter 9, for terminology). The inward background current is almost certainly involved in the early phase of the pacemaker depolarization. However, attempts to reconstruct the full pacemaker potential have shown that, by itself, this current is insufficient to account for all the phenomena observed.

(b) Thus, the reconstruction of pacemaker activity in the Purkinje fibres of the heart (McAllister, Noble, and Tsien 1975) shows that the last phase of the pacemaker depolarization must also depend on a small degree of activation of the sodium current which, when strongly activated, is responsible for the upstroke of the action potential.

(c) However, in the sino-atrial node, the fast sodium current is not significantly involved in pacemaker activity (see Brooks and Lu 1972; Noma and Irisawa 1976a, b; Brown, Giles, and S. J. Noble 1976, 1977b). In this case the second inward (or sodium/calcium) current is involved in the later phase of pacemaker depolarization, as well as in the action potential upstroke.

Under some circumstances it may also be necessary to invoke the contribution of a fourth depolarizing current: the transient inward current observed, for example, in digitalis toxicity (Lederer and Tsien 1976). This component may be important in some forms of heart-rate variability and I shall return to it again later.

One of the important advances in our knowledge of ionic current mechanisms in excitable cells has been the demonstration that each current is formed of small quanta of current flowing through single channels in the cell membrane (see Hille 1970). Some of the statistical properties of the 'noise' generated by the opening and closing of membrane ionic channels have been investigated in recent years (see Verveen and DeFelice 1974). In the case of myelinated nerve it is possible to show that membrane noise may significantly alter the latency of firing of the neuronal spike. An example of this phenomenon is shown in Fig. 2.2.

No systematic study of the role of membrane noise in heart-rate variability has yet been published. There are, however, grounds for thinking that, although such a role is not *a priori* impossible, it is very unlikely from a quantitative point of view.

The rate of depolarization during the pacemaker potential is extremely small, about $20 \, \text{mV s}^{-1}$. Since the ionic current flow is related to the rate of depolarization by the equation

$$i_i = -C\frac{dV}{dt}, \tag{2.1}$$

15

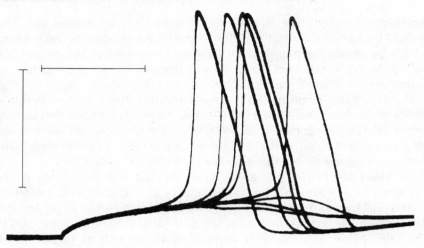

FIG. 2.2. Spontaneous variation in the delay for firing of myelinated nerve during a constant depolarizing current. Calibrations: vertical, 50 mV; horizontal, 1 ms. (Verveen and Derksen 1968.)

where C is the membrane capacity, we can calculate the ionic current involved. Let us consider a mm^2 of membrane in which the membrane capacity will be about $0\cdot01\ \mu F$ (assuming $1\ \mu F\ cm^{-2}$). We then obtain $i = -0\cdot01 \times 10^{-6} \times 0\cdot02\ A = -2 \times 10^{-10}\ A$.

The conductance of a single ionic channel in nerve is about $0\cdot2$ nmho (Hille 1970). If we suppose that the electrical gradient across the channel is about 100 mV (for a sodium channel) we obtain a single-channel current of $0\cdot1 \times 0\cdot2 \times 10^{-9}\ A = 0\cdot2 \times 10^{-10}\ A$, which is not negligible compared to the current calculated as flowing across a mm^2 of membrane during the pacemaker potential. In fact it would be sufficient, if applied to this area of membrane, to change the rate of depolarization by 10 per cent. This calculation suggests that it is not impossible that some random variation in heart-rate might be attributable to single-channel statistical properties. Nevertheless, the ionic current records in Fig. 2.1 do not show very significant noise. This is not, however, surprising since the depolarizing current involved is about $50 \times 10^{-10}\ A$. (This is the net fall in current during a clamp at -60 mV.) The total membrane area involved in the experiment is probably much greater than a mm^2. The crucial question, of course, is over what area would the current supplied by an individual channel be effectively dispersed. A rough estimate for this may be obtained by assuming that the current distributes itself over about a single space constant. In the trabeculae used in obtaining the record shown in Fig. 2.1 the space constant is nearly 1 mm (Brown, Noble, and S. J. Noble 1976). The trabeculae are about 100 μm in width and the individual cells about 5 μm. We will therefore assume that there are of the order of $20 \times 20 = 400$ cells in each cross-section. The total membrane area in a mm of trabeculum will therefore be $2\pi \times 0 \cdot 005 \times 400 \simeq 25$ mm^2. Thus, it is not surprising that the currents flowing are about 25 times larger than would be required in a mm^2 of membrane. These calculations should not be taken too seriously since they are subject to many possible errors, but they do give a rough estimate that allows us to conclude that a single channel current would not, in this case, vary the depolarization rate by more than 0·5 per cent.

It is possible however, that the effective membrane area over which current may flow is considerably smaller in the true sinus or sino-atrial node than it is in the atrial trabeculae used in obtaining records like those of Fig. 2.1. The frog sinus and the mammalian sino-atrial node have recently been studied by voltage clamp methods. The pacemaker currents recorded are not in fact much smaller than in the atrium (see Noma and Irisawa 1976a, b; Brown, Giles, and S. J. Noble 1976, 1977b). At present, therefore, we may conclude that it is not likely that single channel noise contributes significantly to pacemaker variability. This conclusion is further strengthened by the fact that more recent estimates of single channel currents are much smaller than those given by Hille (1970).

Temperature

Another important property of the kinetics of the opening and closing of ionic channels is that a high temperature sensitivity is usually shown. In Purkinje fibres, the Q_{10} for the rate of decay of potassium current during the pacemaker potential can be as high as 17 (Cohen, Daut, and Noble 1976) which means that even quite small variations in temperature may alter the rate of firing (see Weidmann 1956).

This phenomenon is sometimes extremely marked. Fig. 2.3 shows an experiment on rhythmic firing in a sheep Purkinje fibre. These fibres sometimes show pacemaker activity at relatively low membrane potentials and this activity is not dissimilar from that seen in the SA node (see Hauswirth, Noble, and Tsien 1969). In the experiment shown in Fig. 2.3(a), a 3 °C rise in temperature was sufficient to increase the frequency of firing sixfold. Even a 0·1° change in temperature was sufficient to change the firing frequency by 30 per cent.

17

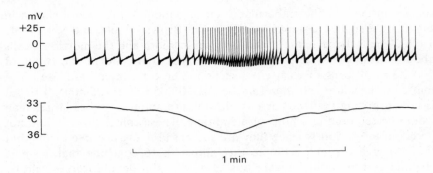

F<small>IG</small>. 2.3. Variation in rate of spontaneous firing in a depolarized Purkinje fibre during a 3° increase in temperature. (Cohen and D. Noble, unpublished.)

2.3. Autonomic transmitters

The natural way in which the heart-rate is controlled by the nervous system is through the release of the autonomic transmitters, acetylcholine, adrenaline, and noradrenaline. The voltage clamp technique has greatly clarified the ionic mechanisms by which this control is effected.

In the case of sympathetic control by adrenergic mechanisms it is now clear that there are important differences between the mechanisms involved in the increase in frequency in different pacemaker tissues. This is so despite the superficial similarity of the pacemaker records during adrenalin action. Fig. 2.4 shows the membrane potential changes during acceleration of (a) the frog sinus and (b) mammalian Purkinje fibre. In both cases the rate of depolarization during the pacemaker potential is increased and the maximum diastolic potential becomes more negative. It should be noted, however, that the pacemaker potentials occur in quite different voltage ranges in the two types of cell. In the sinus the pacemaker range is typically −60 to −40 mV. In Purkinje fibres the range is −90 to −70 mV.

This difference in pacemaker range is reflected in the fact that the potassium current mechanisms involved activate over quite different ranges of potentials (see Brown, McNaughton, D. Noble, and S. J. Noble 1975). In the Purkinje fibre the activation threshold for the pacemaker K^+ current lies at −90 mV and adrenalin accelerates the rate of decay of the current by shifting this threshold in a positive direction (Hauswirth, Noble, and Tsien 1968; Tsien 1974). The reversal potential for the current is also displaced in a negative direction (Cohen, Eisner, and

18

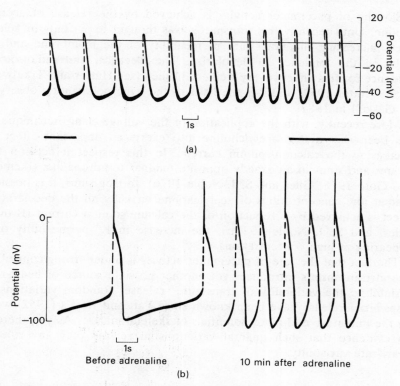

FIG. 2.4. Acceleration of pacemaker activity by sympathetic nerve stimulation and by adrenaline. (a) Frog sinus venosus. The sympathetic nerve was stimulated during break in horizontal line below the voltage trace. (Hutter and Trautwein 1956.) (b) Sheep Purkinje fibre before and after application of adrenaline. (Otsuka 1958.)

D. Noble 1978), probably as a consequence of stimulation of the Na–K exchange pump. This effect accounts for the increase in maximum diastolic potential seen in Fig. 2.4.

In the atrium, the activation threshold for the K^+ current controlling pacemaker activity is about -40 mV and this threshold is *not* changed by adrenalin. Instead, the total amplitude of the current is increased (Brown and S. J. Noble 1974). By itself this effect would slow the rhythm, and the acceleration in this case is attributable to a substantial increase in the second inward (sodium/calcium) current.

19

Slowing of pacemaker activity is achieved by the release of acetyl-choline. Until recently this transmitter was thought to act only by selectively increasing the potassium permeability of the membrane and so reducing the tendency to depolarize. The electrical and radioisotope evidence for this effect is very well established (see Hutter and Trautwein 1956; Hutter 1957) and it is the basis of the hyperpolarization observed by Gaskell in 1887.

More recently, with the application of the voltage clamp technique, it has been shown that acetylcholine also exerts an important effect by decreasing the calcium/sodium current. In this respect it acts on the atrium and sinus in an exactly opposite manner to adrenaline. (Ikemoto and Goto 1975; Giles and S. J. Noble 1976). In frog sinus, it is possible that at low concentrations of acetylcholine virtually all the decelerating effect is achieved by a reduction of the calcium/sodium current (Brown, Giles, and S. J. Noble 1977a), the increase in K^+-permeability only appearing at high concentrations.

The fact that the rate of pacemaker activity is under strong control by neural transmitters introduces yet another possible source of heart-rate variability: the variability of transmitter release. Random variations in transmitter release have been known since Fatt and Katz's (1952) work on the miniature end-plate potentials of skeletal muscle. As yet, there is no evidence that such quantal variations in release play any role in heart-rate variability.

2.4. Cardiac glycosides

Although the membrane currents recorded during voltage clamp experiments of the kind shown in Fig. 2.1 are usually relatively free of noise in healthy preparations, it is well known to workers in this field that as a preparation deteriorates, or while it is still suffering from damage due to dissection, the current records are considerably more noisy.

Recently it has been found possible to induce such noisiness artificially by exposing Purkinje fibres of the mammalian heart to concentrations of cardiac glycoside sufficient to inhibit the sodium–potassium exchange pump. Fig. 2.5 shows the results of an experiment by Lederer and Tsien (1976) using strophanthidin. Each current record shows the decay of pacemaker current. Before administration of glycoside the record is relatively noise-free. Following strophanthidin, the record becomes progressively more noisy. The current mechanism responsible for this effect

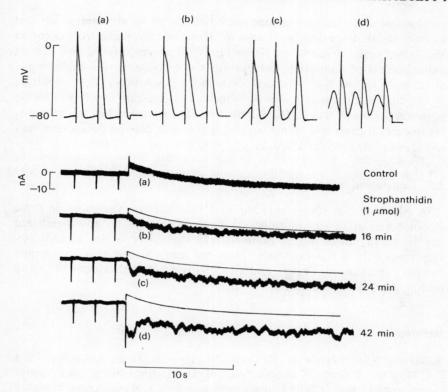

FIG. 2.5. Membrane current variability (noise) induced in Purkinje fibres by strophanthidin. Top records: action potentials before (a) and after (b, c, d) application of strophanthidin. Note development of large spontaneous depolarizations. Bottom records: voltage clamp current records of current decay during pacemaker activity. Note that current variability greatly increases. (Lederer and Tsien 1976.)

has been shown to be responsible for the spontaneous depolarization that may give rise to extra systoles during glycoside toxicity (see Lederer and Tsien 1976).

Is it possible that the glycoside is allowing single-channel noise to become evident in the current records? This is very unlikely. Analysis of the noise involved shows that the unitary event is much larger than would be expected from single-channel currents. It is not yet known what

21

mechanism underlies the current noise introduced by glycosides, nor is it known whether similar enhancement of membrane noise may occur in sino-atrial tissue. Irisawa and Noma (1977), however, have shown that an enhancement of membrane current noise does occur in the rabbit sino-atrial node in low Na^+ solutions, or high Ca^{2+} solutions. The amplitude of the current fluctuation may be sufficient to generate a voltage change between 0·2 and 1·0 mV. The fluctuation was not dependent on transmitter release. Irisawa and Noma suggest that it may depend on spontaneous changes in intracellular calcium.

2.5. Conclusion

In conclusion, it seems very unlikely that random variations in ionic channel activation or transmitter release contribute to any significant degree to the mechanisms of heart-rate variability under normal circumstances. It is however very probable that variability in membrane current mechanisms may underlie arrhythmic behaviour in more pathological circumstances.

References

BANISTER, R. J., BROWN, H. F., GILES, W., HUTTER, O. F., and NOBLE, S. J. (1976). W. H. Gaskell's demonstration of the 'electrical changes in the quiescent cardiac muscle which accompany stimulation of the vagus nerve'. *J. Physiol.* **263**, 60–3P.

BROOKS, C. McC. and LU, M. M. (1972). *The sino-atrial pacemaker of the heart.* Thomas, Springfield, Ill.

BROWN, H. F., CLARK, A., and NOBLE, S. J. (1972). Pacemaker current in frog atrium. *Nature New Biol.* **235**, 30–1.

—— GILES, W., and NOBLE, S. J. (1976). Voltage clamp of frog sinus venosus. *J. Physiol.* **258**, 78–9P.

—— —— —— (1977a). Cholinergic inhibition of frog sinus venosus. *J. Physiol.* **267**, 38–9P.

—— —— —— (1977b). Membrane currents underlying rhythmic activity in frog sinus venosus. *J. Physiol.* **271**, 783–816.

——, McNAUGHTON, P. A., NOBLE, D., and NOBLE, S. J. (1975). Adrenergic control of cardiac pacemaker currents. *Phil. Trans. roy. Soc.* B **270**, 527–37.

—— NOBLE, D., and NOBLE, S. J. (1976). The influence of non-uniformity on the analysis of potassium currents in heart muscle. *J. Physiol.* **258**, 615–29.

—— and NOBLE, S. J. (1974). Effects of adrenaline on membrane currents underlying pacemaker activity in frog atrial muscle. *J. Physiol.* **238**, 51–3P.

COHEN, I., DAUT, J., and NOBLE, D. (1976). The effects of potassium and temperature on the pacemaker current i_{K_2} in Purkinje fibres. *J. Physiol.* **260**, 55–74.

——, EISNER, D., and NOBLE, D. (1978). The action of adrenaline on pacemaker activity in cardiac Purkinje fibres. *J. Physiol.* **280**, 155–68.

DECK, K. A. and TRAUTWEIN, W. (1964). Ionic currents in cardiac excitation. *Pflüger's Arch. ges. Physiol.* **280**, 65–80.

FATT, P. and KATZ, B. (1952). Spontaneous subthreshold activity at motor nerve endings. *J. Physiol.* **117**, 109–28.

GASKELL, W. H. (1883). On the innervation of the heart, with especial reference to the heart of the tortoise. *J. Physiol.* **4**, 43–127.

—— (1887). On the action of muscarin on the heart, and on the electrical changes in the non-beating cardiac muscle brought about by stimulation of the inhibitory and augmentor nerves. *J. Physiol.* **8**, 404–15.

HAUSWIRTH, O., NOBLE, D., and TSIEN, R. W. (1968). Adrenaline: mechanism of action on the pacemaker potential in cardiac Purkinje fibers. *Science* **162**, 916–17.

—— —— —— (1969). The mechanism of oscillatory activity at low membrane potentials in cardiac Purkinje fibres. *J. Physiol.* **200**, 255–65.

HILLE, B. (1970). Ionic channels in nerve membranes. *Prog. Biophys.* **21**, 1–32.

HUTTER, O. F. (1957). Mode of action of autonomic transmitters on the heart. *Br. med. Bull.* **13**, 176–80.

—— and TRAUTWEIN, W. (1956). Vagal and sympathetic effects on the pacemaker fibers in the sinus venosus of the heart. *J. gen. Physiol.* **39**, 715–33.

IKEMOTO, Y. and GOTO, M. (1975). Nature of the negative inotropic effect of acetylcholine on the myocardium. An elucidation on the bullfrog atrium. *Proc. Jap. Acad.* **51**, 501–5.

IRISAWA, H. and NOMA, A. (1977). Miniature fluctuation of the membrane potential in the rabbit sino-atrial node cell. XXVII International Congress of Physiological Sciences, Paris.

LEDERER, W. J. and TSIEN, R. W. (1976). Transient inward current underlying arrythmogenic effects of cardiotonic steroids in Purkinje fibres. *J. Physiol.* **263**, 73–100.

NOBLE, D. (1979). *The initiation of the heartbeat* (2nd edn). Clarendon Press, Oxford.

NOMA, A. and IRISAWA, H. (1976a). Membrane currents in the rabbit sino-atrial node cell as studied by the double microelectrode method. *Pflüger's Arch. ges. Physiol.* **364**, 45–52.

—— —— (1976b). A time- and voltage-dependent potassium current in the rabbit sino-atrial node cell. *Pflüger's Arch. ges. Physiol.* **366**, 251–8.

OTSUKA, M. (1958). Die Virkung von Adrenalin auf Purkinje-fasern von Säugetieren. *Pflügers Arch. ges. Physiol.* **266**, 512–17.

TSIEN, R. W. (1974). Effect of epinephrine on the pacemaker potassium current of cardiac Purkinje fibers. *J. gen. Physiol.* **64**, 293–319.

VERVEEN, A. A. and DeFELICE, J. (1974). Membrane noise. *Prog. Biophys.* **28,** 189–265.

—— and DERKSEN, H. E. (1968). Fluctuation phenomena in nerve membrane. *Proc. IEEE* **56,** 906–16.

WEIDMANN, S. (1956). *Elektrophysiologie der Herzmuskelfaser.* Hans Huber, Bern.

Part II

Techniques of analysis

3.
Signal analysis of heart-rate variability
B. McA. Sayers

THE beat-by-beat variations of heart-rate are neither quite deterministic nor entirely random and, as with most biological variables, successive periods of observation lead to somewhat different results—partly because of the operation of changing biological factors, and partly due to statistical sampling effects. The analysis of heart-rate records must therefore separate the effects of these sources, since interest is almost totally focused on confirming the origins of biological effects, and quantifying these in various interesting situations.

The cardiac signal, in this context, can be regarded as a sequence of point events (occurrences of P or R waves in the ECG) and two types of approach are possible. First, some global features of the point-sequence could be measured. Two such global measures are mean heart-rate and variance of interbeat interval; this kind of measure certainly reflects the existence of changing physiological conditions, but only in a rather unspecific way. It offers a general picture of the interval magnitude about which all intervals cluster, and of the extent of clustering. Such an approach can indicate nothing about any sequential patterns traced out by successive intervals; but, as far as the heart-rate variable is concerned, these patterns offer the only prospect of any detailed picture of the behavior of underlying physiological mechanisms. Thus, a second type of approach is desirable, that studies pattern features of the fluctuations of heart-rate. An analysis which draws on the coherent dynamic features of these fluctuations, rather than on their global description, is potentially more likely to illuminate detailed system structure and properties of the underlying physiological mechanisms: hence the interest in patterns.

3.1. The nature of the heart-rate signal

Long-term properties

The development of ambulatory monitoring techniques made possible the study of heart-rate variations over continuous 24-hour periods both in normal subjects and in patients with cardio-respiratory or other disorders. Normal subjects generate cardiac interbeat interval histograms that are usually skewed rather than Gaussian (especially in day-time records), or that are clearly bimodal (because of respiratory effects, or the existence of two preferred heart-rates). The mean interval, and sometimes also the scatter of intervals, is affected by posture, physical activity, or speaking and other influences on breath pattern. Slow trends that last for periods of up to an hour or more, changing mean heart-rate by as much as 30 per cent, are common in the normal subject, as are sporadic abrupt shifts of rate, or changes in variance. Coherent long-term patterns are rare. Typical interval histograms are shown in Fig. 3.1.

Short-term properties

Pattern aspects are important to the character of the short-term heart-rate record. This can be seen by comparing a sequence of interbeat

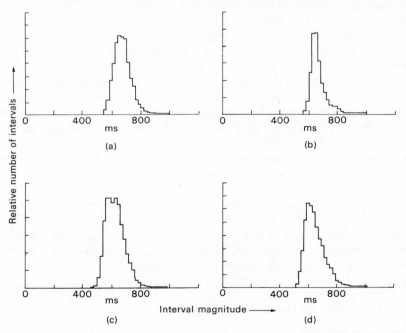

FIG. 3.1. Interbeat interval histograms from a single normal adult subject during a 6-h period, seated and reading for most of the period. A total of about 2000 intervals is included in each record.

28

intervals (i.e. an interval signal) with the same set in randomized, rather than natural, order. In Fig. 3.2(a) and (b), randomization visibly alters the character of the interval signal. Thus the sequence of intervals must be strongly order-dependent; the scatter diagrams (Fig. 3.2(c) and (d)) of the original and randomized sequences, the autocorrelation functions of the two signals (Fig. 3.2(e) and (f)) and their amplitude spectra (Fig. 3.3), all illustrate this clearly. Like the scatter diagrams, the histogram of differences between successive intervals indicates differential effects but cannot directly indicate patterns of relationships between successive intervals, which are responsible for the main features in the autocorrelation function and spectrum of any sequence.

The nature of interrelationships between sequential intervals affects an important statistical property of any sequence of intervals—the degrees of freedom; this can be taken, approximately, to mean the number of independent separate observations contained in any statistical sample. In the heart-rate case, the N-point sequence of successive intervals must comprise rather less than N independent observations. The reason concerns the nature of the autocorrelation function of the interval sequence which, if properly normalized, is, of course, the same function as the serial correlation sequence of intervals.

A sequence of, say, 200 statistically independent intervals can be regarded as a set of 200 independent numbers; all will be needed to represent the record. However, if successive intervals are correlated then, to some extent, later intervals can be predicted from earlier intervals; consequently the set would not necessarily need 200 independent numbers for their complete representation. Indeed, it can be argued that the minimum set of numbers needed fully to represent the fluctuations in the sequence of observations (and this number is quite unrelated to the number required for correct Shannon-sampling of the conceptual 'underlying signal' mentioned below) can be treated as the number of degrees of freedom in that given length of data. It is feasible to estimate experimentally the number of degrees of freedom (DF) per point in the sequence of intervals, from the serial correlation sequence, from the interval power spectrum, or from the standard error of the mean interval if sufficient data are available.

Imagine now that the record–record variations in interval sequences from a given subject could be attributed entirely to statistical sampling effects and not to changing biological factors—a best case assumption. The variability of signal power in successive interval sequences will still be large because of the small number of DF per point: the smaller the DF in

29

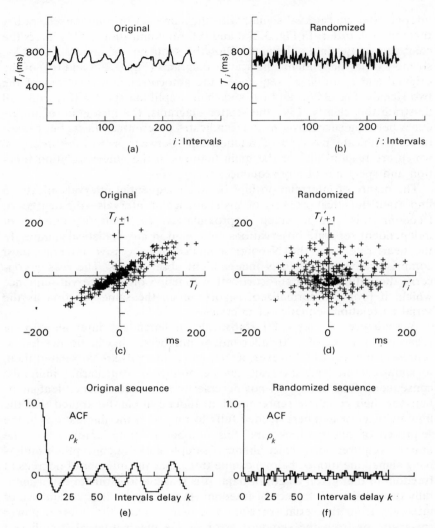

FIG. 3.2. (a) and (b) Original and randomized sequences of successive inter-beat intervals. (c) and (d) Scatter diagrams of successive intervals from the original and from the randomized sequence; the intervals are shown as deviations from the mean interval in each case. The diagram for the original sequence shows clearly the characteristic effect of a recurrent fluctuation in the signal. (e) and (f) Auto-correlation functions (in the form of serial correlation sequences) of the original and of the randomized sequence of intervals.

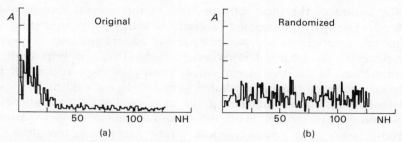

FIG. 3.3. Amplitude spectra for (a) the original and (b) randomized sequences of 256 sequential intervals; NH is harmonic number, NH = 1 representing 1 cycle per 256 intervals. Randomization converts the sequence into a statistical sample from a random source and, apart from statistical sampling fluctuations, the spectrum is then constant.

a record, the larger the statistical sampling variations. When the already limited number of DF in the record are shared amongst a few, possibly independent, spectral bands, the situation is much worse. This is the reason for the large variability of the spectral density of interval signal power, for which the coefficient of variation may be about unity (see below and Fig. 3.6). Typical values for DF per point are $0 \cdot 1$–$0 \cdot 2$ but these can alter with sample length when long lengths of data are involved because of non-stationarity of the mean or variance.

Since the effects due to statistical variability in the interval signal are substantial they are very likely to mask any effects due to biological factors, for example the effect of information work-load on the subject (during a perceptual-loading task). The only way to cope with this kind of difficulty is to compile more data in some way—either by increasing the record length or, where this is appropriate, by forming an ensemble of responses to some specific imposed load. The former is likely to be difficult in the experimental laboratory (although both realistic and appropriate in the analysis of spontaneous heart-rate variability under clinical conditions), but the ensemble analysis approach is practically effective, even across subjects.

Sequential relationships can also be explored to some extent by examining the event-autocorrelation—also known as expectation density (Sayers 1970)—of the point-event signal. However the only really useful indications that result lie in broad features of the function: specifically, the presence of non-stationarity in the process; this produces visible 'beats' of the periodicities in the function and directs attention to the need for segmentation of the record.

31

The nature of the short-term patterns in the interval record, which reflects underlying biological processes, is clarified by separating the signal into components, say, according to any evident grouping of spectral components. As discussed elsewhere, Sayers (1973), it is possible to confirm that, in the short-term signal, activity in three regions of the interval spectrum can be attributed substantially to explicit biological origins—in respiratory movement, in quasi-oscillatory fluctuations of blood-pressure associated with the dynamic control of mean arterial blood-pressure, and in slower, more erratic fluctuations thought to be associated with thermal regulation (by adjustments of superficial blood-flow).

There are three approaches to the analysis of heart-rate records. Traditional statistical methods can be applied to the set of interbeat interval magnitudes. The interval sequence, or some set of values derived from it, can be treated as a signal, and the usual methods of signal analysis then applied. Finally, when coherent patterns are likely to occur in the records, pattern analysis methods may be employed to identify and quantify pattern features: the most likely occasion for pattern analysis occurs in the study of stimulated responses.

3.2. Statistical techniques of analysis

Choice of variables

Three discrete variables related to heart-rate suggest themselves: interbeat interval, beat-by-beat rate (the reciprocal of interval), and the count of beats in a specific period of time. For statistical reasons argued in Cox and Lewis (1966) and also discussed in Sayers (1970, 1973), the interval statistics are basic in that many of the count- and rate-statistics can be derived from them.

Statistical moments

Subject to the requirements for stationarity (discussed below), the mean interval and the variance, or the standard deviation, of intervals can, of course, be easily estimated from the data. In practice, however, it is necessary to remember the effects of length-biased sampling of intervals, and to consider the accuracy of any calculations carried out in a digital computer of limited precision. Length-bias effects only arise if intervals are selected randomly by arbitrary instant (measuring the magnitude of the interval then current), and this situation is unlikely to be met, though possible, in the context of estimating moments of distribution. But appreciable errors can occur in calculating mean and variance, especially with a large sample, and a method due to Stagg largely circumvents the problem. If D is the difference between the new data value x_n and the mean for all previous values (m_{n-1}) then

$$m_n = m_{n-1} - D/n \quad \text{with} \quad D = m_{n-1} - x_n,$$

while if B_{n-1} is $(n-2)$ times the variance up to the $(n-1)$th term, the variance for the first n terms can be calculated

$$S_n^2 = \frac{B_n}{n-1} \quad \text{with} \quad B_n = B_{n-1} + \frac{(n-1)D^2}{n}.$$

These calculations can be carried out iteratively and efficiently; the method can be generalized to the calculation of running covariance and running correlation coefficient.

Higher order moments can also be calculated directly from the data in a corresponding way. However if the histogram is multimodal it may be better to carry out the calculations on the (smoothed) histogram since then the separate components can probably be individually quantified, provided the modal separation is sufficient.

Estimating degrees of freedom

This parameter, DF, can be expressed conveniently as DF per point, by dividing the total DF estimated for a given sample size by the number of data points it contains. The DF appropriate to mean values of a variable, indicating the variability of its sample mean, can be estimated by calculating across many trials the ensemble average standard error $\overline{SE}_N$ of the mean of the given sample size N, and deducing DF_N from it. The DF-figure appropriate to estimates of signal power or signal spectrum, indicating their likely variability, is calculable from the ensemble average discrete spectral density of the signal power across various members of an ensemble of signal lengths—i.e. samples of variable. The two measures only coincide in the case of a constant spectral density signal—when the total power in the signal is distributed uniformly over the spectral band. However they are often comparable. (The variability of the sample mean of a stationary random variable can be shown (Bendat and Piersol 1966) to involve an integral measure of the autocorrelation function. In the case of signal power estimates, the squared autocorrelation function also enters the integral.) Since the signal spectrum describes a resolution of

33

the total signal power into individual components or bands, the appropriate DF-figure to be resolved into the contributions from the corresponding spectral bands is therefore that of signal power. Thus, we now consider the procedures for estimating the two DF measures.

If the population standard deviation σ_e of cardiac interval can be estimated with precision from a large sample of intervals, then for a specified sample size N the estimated standard error SE_N of the sample mean for samples of size N is given by $\sigma_e/(DF)^{\frac{1}{2}}$. The standard error can be determined empirically by calculating the observed SD of the means of many samples of the pre-determined size N; then $DF_N = (\sigma_e/\overline{SE}_N)^2$.

Estimates of standard deviation (SD), and of standard error (SE_N) for samples of length N, both tend to increase with record length due to the unavoidable non-stationarities. The SD estimate alters because changes in the long-term mean value increases the 'offset' of earlier parts of the record; the SE_N alters because the means of successive N-point samples tend to fluctuate if influenced by the non-stationarity. In a number of cases it has been confirmed that these effects are relatively more important in the case of SE_N; but in either variable the matter of defining a 'true' mean value is not trivial.

For these reasons it is best to compromise by segmenting the record into lengths within which slow non-stationarities due to long-term effects are generally small. The DF per point can then be estimated by forming the squared ratio of the SD to SE_N estimates for a sufficient ensemble of these record lengths (each N_R) where the sample size N is chosen so as to include a reasonable number (say 8) of samples in the basic record length N_R. The ensemble mean of DF per point is used, preferably calculated from the best single estimates of σ_e and SE_N.

The choice of sample size, N, in this case is influenced by short-term non-stationarities in the record—particularly by pattern features in the record. For example, if the pattern happens to comprise several fluctuations with roughly constant period, then samples that cover about half this period, if taken contiguously (as often necessary in this kind of analysis for practical reasons), would experience maximum change in the mean from one sample to the next. The squared ratio of apparent SD to SE_N will then produce unrealistic values of DF and so, DF per point.

The detailed pattern of the record, say a sequence of $N_R = 256$ intervals, will be influenced by the phase spectrum which, however, will not affect the serial correlation or the power spectrum of the record; hence the phase spectrum is irrelevant to the DF per point. So, reconstituting the signal with the same amplitude (and power) spectrum but various phase spectra (e.g. determined from a table of random numbers uniformly distributed over the principal-angle range) produces an ensemble of signals with different patterns, but unaltered serial correlation and power spectrum, and so, unaltered expected value of DF per point. But the DF per point estimated from the squared ratio of SD/SE$_N$ will fluctuate with sample size N in a somewhat different way each time, in accordance with the apparent non-stationarity occasioned by the broad features of individual pattern in the record. Averaged over a sufficient range of patterns, however, the DF per point estimated in this way should and does approximate a realistic value.

This matter can be illuminated somewhat by showing the effect of phase modification of an ensemble of interval sequences, as shown in Fig. 3.4. A 10-member original ensemble is shown, on the left. Each record is reconstituted into a new signal having the amplitude spectrum of the original but random phase in successive harmonics; these new signals are shown in the centre of Fig. 3.4. (If the same random phase pattern is used for each record, thus allowing only the amplitude spectrum to alter each time, the reconstitution produces the ensemble on the right side of Fig. 3.4; the similarities under the influence of this phase constraint are appreciable.) New short-term patterns are thus created by this phase adjustment. Each of these three ensembles gives a spectrally-based estimate of 0·17 DF per point but the squared ratio of SD to SE$_N$ produces results that are sample-size dependent (varying from 0·08 to 0·28 in a slightly different way according to pattern) but again averaging out at 0·17 over a variety of trials.

Such estimates of degrees of freedom are useful in various ways. Traditionally, of course, they clarify the extent of improvement of confidence limits with sample size on estimates of mean interval. But it must be remembered that if the requirement for independence of successive samples is violated (by considering contiguous samples) then local pattern fluctuations may act like non-stationarities and cause substantial increases in the estimated standard error of the mean interval.

More important uses for degrees of freedom estimates are frequently met. In patient surveillance, for example, it would be necessary to test if the short-term mean interval is significantly altered from earlier values; additionally a second key question might be if the power or the spectral pattern of intervals, say, had changed beyond the typical spontaneous limits. In the first case the appropriate DF of the data is the first-order DF describing the mean interval. In the second case, the appropriate DF would need to be extracted for the relevant spectral band from the

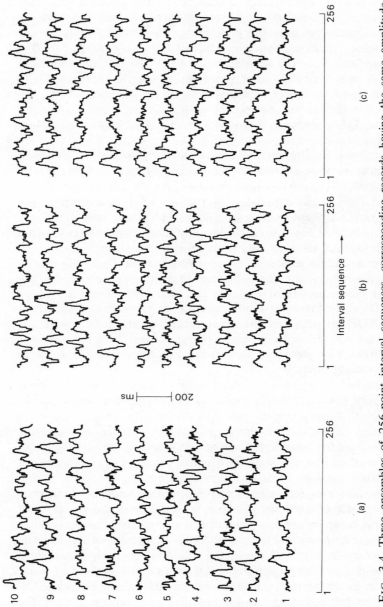

Fig. 3.4. Three ensembles of 256-point interval sequences, corresponding records having the same amplitude spectrum, autocorrelation function, and estimated degrees of freedom. The original ensemble (a) was obtained from a resting subject. The other ensembles were reconstructed from the original using, for corresponding records, the original amplitude spectrum; the ensemble (b) used randomized phases for each harmonic, but the same set of random phases was used for all the individual records in ensemble (c).

second-order (power) DF. In both cases, if a suitable statistical measure can be devised, the appropriate DF value would be required.

A more tricky application also occurs—in the detection of coherent average responses that may have unexpected or unpredictable pattern features. Testing a given result for the presence of an explicit pattern can be based merely on a statistical discrimination of the extreme magnitudes of the signal. But the complete pattern might be tested instead, by comparing pre-stimulus signal power or spectrum with the post-stimulus signal. The appropriate DF measures are again needed, in conjunction with some estimates of the probability density function of the variable being tested. (Because of the difficulties of this approach, Sayers and Beagley introduced an objective test for responses, based on the phase-spectral statistics of the post-stimulus record, using the phase correlate of a response pattern (Sayers, Beagley, and Rhia 1979); however this has only been used in EEG responses so far.)

The second DF measure can be estimated by a method discussed by Bendat and Piersol (1966), based on an approach due to Blackman and Tukey (1958) and outlined in Sayers (1975b). It depends on estimating the discrete spectrum of interval signal power generated by the hypothesized underlying signal source (it is necessary to ensemble average the smoothed discrete spectral power due to a number of signal samples). Then the DF of the random Gaussian white-noise signal having the same statistical variability of the power is estimated by

$$\mathrm{DF}_e = 2\left(\sum_1^M P_i\right)^2 \bigg/ \sum_1^M P_i^2,$$

where $M = N/2$, and P_i is the power (squared amplitude) of the ith Fourier harmonic, obtained from the smoothed ensemble-average of the discrete power spectrum. It will be recognized that this formulation assesses the variation of the spectrum from constancy and so, indirectly, the deviation of the autocorrelation function from a Dirac pulse form; either situation implies serial correlation of sample values, some predictability of later values from earlier values, and reduced DF.

The value for DF in the case of power estimates can be used to indicate the likely variability of power in records of the specified length (i.e. in samples of the specified size). It would also be used in significance testing of power changes between different experimental conditions, including those for which coherent averaging is appropriate (i.e. when the change results in a definable pattern). In addition, it would be this kind of DF that is needed for describing variability of signal power in different

37

spectral bands, the DF being then calculated from the profile of the ensemble-averaged power spectrum in the band concerned.

Non-stationarity

The implication of time-independence of statistical parameters, in the underlying population from which individual sample records are drawn, is quite central to further statistical analysis. It can be tested by non-parametric Trend test (Bendat and Piersol 1966) in the case of single fixed-length interval sequences. But if continuous testing is required, then trend function methods, like the Brown–Trigg approach, can be used.

The Trend test is carried out, using each sequential interval value in turn as a reference, by determining the total number of reverse-arrangements (values higher placed in the sequence than the reference that are nevertheless smaller in magnitude than the reference), and using tables for significance testing of the result.

The Brown–Trigg approach uses an exponentially weighted sum of past interval values (achieved by a simple auto-regressive calculation) as a forecast of future values; at each point the forecasting error is obtained and a tracking-signal is calculated from the ratio of the low-pass filtered error signal and the smoothed rectified error. For a signal of known statistics (e.g. Gaussian) the probability level at which a trend is recognized is related in a specific known way to the tracking signal (Brown 1962; Trigg 1964; Lewis 1971).

If the data sequence is x_k $(k = 1, 2, ...)$, the forecast value based on information available at point k is $\hat{x}_k$, the error signal is e_k, and the smoothed error and smoothed absolute deviation of the error are SMER_k and SMAD_k respectively, then

forecast: $\hat{x}_k = \alpha x_k + (1 - \alpha)\hat{x}_{k-1}$

error in forecast: $e_k = x_k - \hat{x}_{k-1}$

smoothed error; $\mathrm{SMER}_k = \mu e_k + (1 - \mu)\mathrm{SMER}_{k-1}$

smoothed mean absolute deviation: $\mathrm{SMAD}_k = \mu|e_k| + (1 - \mu)\mathrm{SMAD}_{k-1}$

where α and μ are constants. The judged presence of a trend is based on the value of tracking signal

$$\mathrm{TS}_k = \frac{\mathrm{SMER}_k}{\mathrm{SMAD}_k}.$$

$\mathrm{TS} = \pm 1$ corresponds to complete certainty of a positive or negative trend, and the cumulative probability table can be determined in practice for the variable by observations on an adequate sequence of representative stationary intervals. The smoothing parameter α should be chosen small enough that the natural low-frequency fluctuations of the data sequence of (intervals) do not mask the presence of any developing trend that would constitute a non-stationarity which may be significant in itself or perhaps merely inconvenient for statistical reasons, if undetected. Random sources, or the activity of various underlying physiological processes (respiratory or autonomic, for example) could originate such a non-stationarity. The smaller α the longer the filter 'settling' time and the slower any indication of a real trend would develop. The parameter μ should be chosen small enough to prevent these spontaneous fluctuations from causing the tracking signal to reach the confidence level for the presence of a trend. Values of $\alpha = 0\cdot02$ and $\mu = 0\cdot03$ have been found suitable for use in the cardiac interbeat interval sequence; the start-up run of the system is then about 65 points (Thai Thien Nghia 1977).

An example of trend detection using the Brown–Trigg procedure appears in Fig. 3.5: a set of cardiac intervals is shown in which a generally linear trend is present. The interval sequence is stationary in respect of any periods extending about 50 intervals, but a linear trend has been added, starting at point 200 and continuing to point 450, with a slope of $0\cdot5$ ms/interval, or about $0\cdot01$ σ/interval in this record. The trend actually employed was extracted from the same subject, later in time than the resting record used for the interval sequence, and added into the resting interval sequence. The tracking signal (TS) is shown, and the 95-per cent confidence levels for the existence of a trend are also indicated. This kind of analysis also allows the statistics of the occurrences and durations of non-stationarities to be determined.

The above tests mainly pertain to the mean-value parameter, but can, of course, be adapted to the SD or variance as well. While mean interval and SD are sometimes linked, it is possible for the interval SD to alter without affecting the mean interval significantly. One example is due to a change in the pattern of breathing, or to a period of speech which, through the mechanism of sinus arrhythmia, affects the scatter of interbeat intervals, but not necessarily the mean.

The nature of any non-stationarity should dictate its treatment as well as indicating possible origins for its existence that can be explored. If it is of a slowly-varying monotonic kind, trend removal can be carried out. If it produces unpredictable and sporadic effects, then records would be segmented and analysed further in groups according to the range of values exhibited by the parameter.

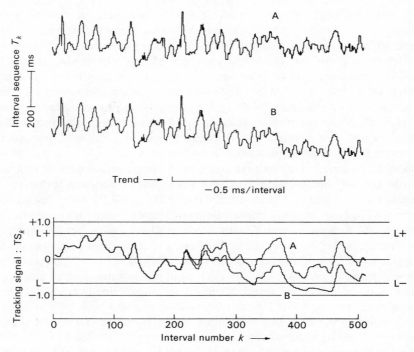

FIG. 3.5. Detection of a linear trend by Brown–Trigg constant parameter tracking-signal analysis. The upper trace shows (A) an original 512-point interval sequence, and (B) the same sequence with added linear trend as indicated (approximately −0·5 ms/interval from intervals 200 to 450, obtained as described in text). The two lower traces show the tracking signals for the two sequences. That for A remains within the 95 per cent confidence levels (L+ and L−) for detection of a trend; that for B is sustained outside the confidence band from interval 384 to 462. These tracking signals show the start-up performance of the system and its responses to typical, if large, slow spontaneous fluctuations, as well as to a short-lasting monotonic trend.

3.3. Signal measures

Choice of signal

Signal analysis of a point-event sequence can be carried out, in principle, in three ways: by focusing on the point sequence in event, count, or interval terms. As an event signal the instants of occurrence are indicated by a standardized event such as a Dirac pulse: the resulting signal is

40

treated as continuous in the time domain. This approach has proved to have relatively little to recommend it for the present purpose. Count-measures depend on representing the point sequence in terms of rate, but despite the attractiveness of thus having a physiologically relevant vari-able, much of the resulting statistical information turns out to be merely a transformation of various interval-statistical measures, Sayers (1970). Consequently interval measures are treated as basic to the representation and analysis of heart-rate variability: analytical descriptions such as the serial correlation of intervals, the interval spectrum, and the band-filtered version of the interval sequence, are all useful.

Nevertheless, it is widely assumed that the cardiac event or interval sequence can be associated with, or attributed to, a continuous underlying signal. This notion and its implications need some brief examination. The effect of the assumption is that any such underlying signal could, and should for various purposes commonly regarded as important, be sampled regularly in the time-domain. In practice, this regularization of the sequence of samples turns out to be entirely unimportant (except perhaps in one situation, namely when it is required to compare the cardiac signal with some simultaneous ongoing waveform, such as mean arterial blood pressure, with reasonably high precision.)

This model of the process regards the interval magnitudes, or the cycle by cycle heart rate, as a set of discrete irregular samples of some underlying continuous waveform which purports to reflect the integrated autonomic activity converging on the sino-atrial node. To regularize the equivalent samples, it is usual to set up each interval magnitude at the instant of termination of that interval. This produces a series of irregular, variable-height samples which purport to represent the underlying inter-val 'signal' at the instants of successive heartbeats. Passing each sample magnitude through a 'zero-order hold' maintains the signal at this level until new information is obtained from the arrival of the next interval magnitude. The low-pass filtered version of this signal will then produce a smooth continuous waveform which can be resampled regularly in the time domain.

However, if this model is regarded as acceptable, it is necessary to answer one critical specific question, namely: is the average sampling rate of the underlying signal (which rate is determined entirely by the mean heart rate) adequate to avoid aliasing? This can only be answered indirectly, perhaps by looking at the spectrum of the hypothesized under-lying waveform to see whether the amplitude of various spectral compo-nents falls off sufficiently rapidly near the highest frequency set by the effective Nyquist rate. Results suggest that a mean heart-rate distinctly above $100\,\text{min}^{-1}$ may be required to avoid significant aliasing. At lower rates, there will thus be unpredictably large errors at unpredictable times in this signal; any high-frequency pattern information may be unusable.

Pre-processing

Since the most convenient signal processing methods involve frequency domain operations, the so-called leakage of signal power into unwanted neighbouring frequencies must be avoided. This can be achieved by removing any linear trend, as estimated by a linear regression, and tapering the resultant down to the mean value over, say, the first and last 10 per cent of the data length. Also, if auto- or cross-correlation operations are to be carried out by frequency domain operations, then the decision must be made if the length of data is to stand alone, or if it can be imagined to link back on itself as if periodic. In the former case the data length (trend and mean removed, tapered) must be followed by an equal length of zero values to generate a 'non-circular' correlation. In the latter case, a 'circular' correlation is acceptable and the added zeros are unnecessary.

Variability analysis

It is sometimes desirable to test if a number of sequential lengths of cardiac interval data can be thought of as generated by a homogeneous source, or if some extraneous factor is sometimes operative to influence the character of the signal. The same question might be asked about the spontaneous signals obtained from a number of subjects immediately prior to some stimulus-response experiment.

One technique is to estimate the degrees of freedom in the individual signal from the average power spectrum of the ensemble of signals (as above) and then to compare the result with the DF calculated as before from the variability of signal power; significant differences between the two DF estimates indicates inhomogeneity within the ensemble. If the amplitude histogram of intervals is gaussian then the comparison can be made through the coefficient of variation $CV = (2/DF)^{\frac{1}{2}}$ which estimates the ratio of SD/mean of the a.c. power values, one for each member of the ensemble; again, the empirical figures can be obtained from the ensemble average and ensemble standard deviation of the a.c. power in the individual signal (Sayers 1975*b*).

A knowledge of the distribution of total a.c. power in the signal, and of the variability of the spectral distribution of the power, is crucial to detecting and quantifying changes in the heart-rate signal by means of spectral descriptions. If the signal were completely random and gaussian distributed then the instantaneous a.c. power might be expected to distribute as χ^2 (1 degree of freedom), while the total a.c. power in a record comprising a substantial number of intervals would be gaussian, and the individual harmonic power would be distributed as χ^2 (2 DF) i.e. in a negative-exponential manner. While these expectations would apply for a signal-like stationary random Gaussian white noise, they are also approximately met in the cardiac interbeat interval case. Fig. 3.6 illustrates the extent of the power spectral variations that are met in the analysis of heart-rate records from a single individual in the resting state.

Spectral analysis and frequency-domain operations

Spectral analysis would be justified if it produced a compact, quantitative representation of a more complex set of numbers (intervals, or some related measure), or if it drew attention to or emphasized some important contributory components. Regardless of the significance of the signal spectrum however, frequency-domain operations are useful in their own right to allow other analyses to be achieved efficiently. Of these, band-selective filtering, correlational operations, and some non-linear processes like complex demodulation are often effected through frequency-domain manipulations.

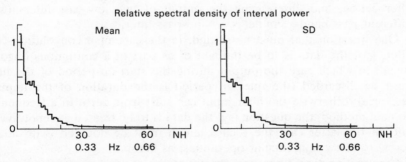

FIG. 3.6. Variability of the smoothed spectral density estimate of the interval signal power in 25 128-interval lengths of signal from one resting subject. The mean spectral power density and its standard deviation are shown to the same scale for each relevant harmonic component (frequency in Hz is also shown). Note that the coefficient of variation (SD/mean of the power) is approximately 1·0, indicating the extremely large variability.

The basic numerical operation used in Fourier spectral calculations is the fast-Fourier transform (FFT). This imposes some limits on the data lengths (most commonly to a power of 2), which may be inconvenient. In this case, the Chirp-Z transform of general length can be used. (Monro 1975, 1976, 1977; Monro and Branch 1977).

It is usually presumed that the emergence of specific patterns in the heart-rate or interval record (for example, pressure vasomotor oscillations with about a 10-s period) would be indicated by an increase of spectral amplitudes over the relevant spectral range. But patterns in the record may also originate in time-synchronization of activity, which could result only in a change in the phase spectrum without any corresponding change in amplitude spectrum. Naturally, in the interval signal the appearance of any (say) oscillatory burst in the record is arbitrarily located with respect to the start of the record, and the phase spectrum will include a time-delay contribution from this source; further, wrap-around effects (the principal angle range of phase is ±180°) additionally complicate the phase spectrum. These matters need to be taken into account when the interpretation of phase spectra is undertaken. The importance of phase is also demonstrated in Fig. 3.4.

Band-selective filtering therefore must not alter phase relationships within the passband—hence the need for zero-phase-shift filters, which can be implemented either by convolution operations or completely in the frequency domain. In either case the output of a zero-phase-shift, low-pass filter can be subtracted from the input record to produce a high-pass filter action, and differencing the output of two low-pass filters (with different pass bands) simulates a band-pass filter.

One question that must be settled, in the case of a convolution-type filter, is if the data is to be thought of as part of a continuous ongoing signal, in which case the output during the start-up-period of the filter must be discarded (the relevant period is the duration of the impulse response); otherwise the filter input can start from zero. In a frequency-domain method, the question is if the data is to be treated as repetitive or not. In the latter case the record length must be doubled (with added zeros) to allow non-circular operations, as before.

Convolution-type filters are strictly of the moving-average type; each new output value y_n is formed as the sum of weighted (a_k) earlier input values x_{n-k}:

$$y_n = \sum_{k=-N}^{+N} a_k x_{n-k}.$$

The profile of the a_k specifies the impulse response of the filter. A much more efficient approach is to utilize some previous output values in the calculation of new values; a simple example is the negative exponential weighting:

$$y_n = (1-a)y_{n-1} + ax_n$$

Details of useful designs can be found in Lynn (1977).

Band-selective filtering. The patterns of activity in the interval signal due to various linearly additive effects can be clarified to a limited extent by band-selective filtering. For example, attending to so-called thermal, pressure vasomotor, and respiratory components in a sequence of, say, 256 successive intervals, the appropriate band-selective filters would transmit the first 10 or so harmonics (H1–H10) of the fundamental Fourier component (1 cycle/256 intervals, or about 1 cycle/200 s = 0·005 Hz at a sample mean interval of 800 ms), H15–H30, and, say, H35–H100, with suitable tapering of the edges of each band. These would, in principle, select the 'thermal' activity, the 'pressure-vasomotor' activity if present, and the respiratory contribution respectively. But the matter is not quite so simple.

Respiratory activity is often rather irregular, especially when the subject is concentrating on some difficult mental work-load task, and as a result the pattern of its effect is then very broadly distributed over the interval spectrum. Indeed, it is noticeable that in these circumstances there is sometimes a distinct shift in the signal power attributable to respiratory activity down towards the pressure-vasomotor band; but since this reflects a particular pattern of respiratory behaviour there are strong inter-subject differences of detail. However, if respiratory behaviour is central, then other methods of measurement would be appropriate (Sayers 1975a).

So-called 'pressure-vasomotor' activity is, in some ways, more difficult to detect and quantify, for reasons that have been discussed elsewhere (Hyndman, Kitney, and Sayers 1971; Hyndman 1974; Sayers 1973). Briefly, this activity takes the form of a relatively broad-band oscillation that appears in bursts of just a few cycles (period 8–12 s), recurring quite irregularly, sometimes with intervals of 5 min or more. The active phase may include from 2–3 cycles up to 25 or more—and, in the former situation, the fact that the activity looks like a truncated oscillation means that there is a wide-band spread of spectral power due to this oscillation. Band-selective filtering thus does not produce an improved representation of the oscillation.

Fig. 3.7 illustrates (in (i)) a 256-interval sequence and its low-frequency filtered version. These low-frequency components have no very definite oscillatory frequency; in so far as any individual oscillation can even be identified, this would be recognized as subject to appreciable and relatively rapid frequency shifts (see below). The band-selected version (ii) shows the H25–H64 band-filtered interval signal and the fluctuations can be shown to follow somewhat (not always proportionately) the thoracic movements of breathing. Close examination shows that this selectively emphasized respiratory sinus arrhythmia can be identified in the raw data (after removal of the mean interval, as in (iv)). Finally the H15–H25 band filtered signal should emphasize any pressure vasomotor oscillations when present. In this record there are perhaps two periods of such oscillation: from interval 1 to about 50, and from about interval 75 to 150 (which can be explored in detail by complex demodulation if necessary). Again the activity can be observed in the raw data (iv).

Fig. 3.8 shows another band-filtered record (i) which can be used conveniently to clarify some of the problems of interpreting spectra. There are several bursts of so-called pressure-vasomotor activity in this record, and for our present purposes these can be extracted separately, and individually embedded in zeros up to a length of 256 intervals again as shown in (ii) and (iv), or jointly as in (iii). The amplitude and phase spectra of the Fig. 3.8(ii) and (iv) records are shown in Fig. 3.9(a) and 3.9(b) respectively, curves i and ii. In each case, over the range of high amplitude components from H12 to 20 and 22 to 25 (Fig. 3.9(a)) and H12 to 27 (Fig. 3.9(b)), the phase spectrum is complicated and uninformative; the significance of the amplitude spectrum is, nevertheless, quite clear. However, optimally spinning the signal on its time base (of 256 intervals) to locate the active segment at its most nearly symmetrical position with respect to the start of the record, simplifies the relevant part of the phase spectrum completely. The result is shown in curves (iv) of Fig. 3.9(a) and (b) for the two separate segmental signals, and in each case phase spectrum over the relevant band represents essentially the pattern of the signal waveform itself, freed from the phase contribution of signal location along the time base and the wrap-around effects that confuse the result. Since the two signals (Fig. 3.8(ii) and (iv)) share many spectral components, this combination (Fig. 3.8(iii)) has an amplitude spectrum in (Fig. 3.9(c)(i)) which is appreciably more complex than either because of the relative phases of corresponding components (sometimes largely adding, sometimes largely subtracting). This is the reason why it is sometimes difficult to recognize the existence of such components through their spectral representation.

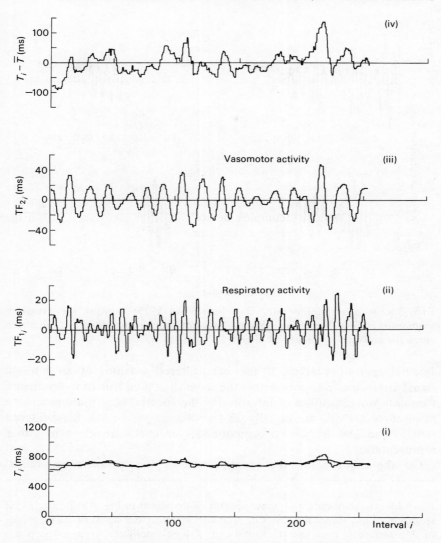

FIG. 3.7. A 256-point cardiac interval sequence (i) superimposed with its low-pass filtered version (d.c. + harmonics (H) 1–5 plus a 5-harmonic taper down to zero transmission). The pattern of fluctuations around the sample mean is shown in (iv). The curves (ii) and (iii), respectively, result from band-filtering the record from H25 to H64 and H15 to 25 respectively, in each case with a 5-harmonic taper at each end of the passband.

47

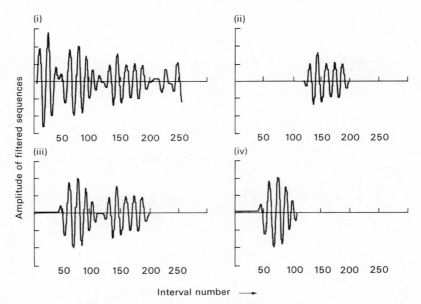

FIG. 3.8. A band-filtered interval sequence (H15–25) showing the pressure-vasomotor activity (i) and two separate bursts of activity embedded individually in zeros (ii) and (iv), or jointly as in (iii).

Interval spectral analysis. If the band-filtered versions of an interval signal are instructive, presumably the same should be true of its spectrum. Certainly the difficulties of interpreting the spectral contributions due to respiratory activity are equally as troublesome as in the band-filtered signal. The low frequency components, however, are clear in either representation.

On the other hand, the identification of the 'pressure-vasomotor'

FIG. 3.9.(a) Amplitude and phase spectra of the signal in Fig. 3.8(ii). The phase spectrum of (iv) shows the result of optimally spinning the signal on its time base of 256-intervals; over the relevant band of high-amplitude spectra, the phase spectrum has assumed a simple readily comprehensible form because of the elimination of added time delay phase shift with consequent phase wrap-around problems. (b) Amplitude and phase spectra for the original (i, ii) signal of Fig. 3.8(iv), and after optimal spinning (in (iii), (iv)). (c) The amplitude and phase spectrum for the combined signal of Fig. 3.8(iii), showing the complication of the amplitude spectrum due to the combination of common spectral components.

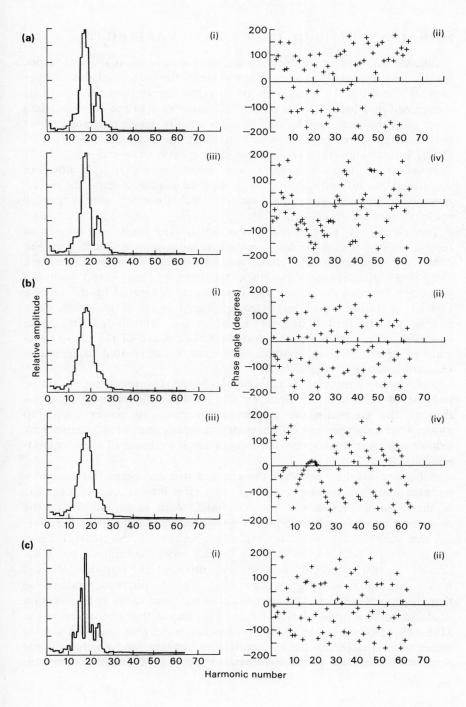

Harmonic number

oscillation is, surprisingly enough, distinctly equivocal in spectral terms, for a rather important reason. When present, the pattern of this component of the interval signal, with all its typical properties, can often be recognized in a band-filtered record but not always in the corresponding spectrum. The fact that the oscillation is usually active only for a short period within a record means that its spectrum is quite widely-spread. Closer investigation then reveals that some lengths of record in which the component is evidently present, and others in which it is not, are sometimes not noticeably different in their amplitude spectra; the differences only emerge in their phase spectra which are much more difficult to interpret (see above and Fig. 3.4).

This aspect can be confirmed in a simple way using two lengths of record, one of which exhibits the 'pressure-vasomotor' oscillation, the other not. Amplitude and phase spectra of the two records are then computed, interchanged (amplitude spectrum of one linked with the phase spectrum of the other) and new signals generated by the inverse Fourier operation. Each reconstructed signal is found to match quite closely the particular original signal which contributed its phase spectrum—thus illustrating the dominant importance of the phase spectrum in determining the pattern which can be attributed to pressure-vasomotor activity.

Unfortunately therefore it must be concluded that it may not always be possible to recognize the presence of 'pressure-vasomotor' oscillations through the interval-signal amplitude spectrum (or power spectrum) alone. Certainly there is no guarantee that any individual record may exhibit any clear amplitude- or power-spectral evidence of these components.

A further difficulty concerns the changes that can occur in respiratory patterns with, say, mental-work load, and their interactions with activity in the 'pressure-vasomotor' spectral band. With some individuals the onset of a mental work-load task is associated with a change in respiratory rate such that its cardiac interval effect approaches the spectral region of the 'pressure-vasomotor' activity. In this band the additive combination of the two signal contributions (regardless of any non-linearity that may exist) will produce a resultant that is highly phase-dependent—so that the power (and spectral amplitude) in the band could either increase or decrease as a result of this change. This means that alterations in the H15–H30 spectral region of the cardiac interval signal might be due to either of two different causes (respiratory changes, and changes in the amount or extent of 'pressure-vasomotor' activity). Distinctly ambiguous spectral changes can occur: different individuals may exhibit quite different (perhaps opposite) effects. One useful aspect of spectral analysis is that it may allow confirmation that the signal can be distinguished from white noise, over a specific frequency band.

This might be thought desirable in respect of low-frequency spectral components, supposedly attributable to 'thermal' physiological activity. The procedure is to test the null hypothesis of a flat spectrum over the band (say, H1–H10 of 1 cycle/256 intervals as before); the most common method is based on a Kolmogorov–Smirnov test, which utilizes cumulative statistics and, like the χ^2-method, tests the differences between the hypothesized and observed curves of (cumulative) spectral power of the a.c. power—normalized record. Maximum error is checked against tabulated significance levels (Siegel 1956). Fig. 3.10 shows the analysis with a single record. The critical level for $P = 0.05$ using the hypothesis of a uniform power spectral density is also indicated; the cumulative power curve does not cross the limit values. Thus in this particular record of 1024 intervals, non-uniformity of this part of the spectrum is not suggested.

Elucidating non-linear effects

Short period variations in either the amplitude or frequency of any explicit oscillatory component in a signal is a non-linear effect. This is met most evidently in the apparent variations of the so-called pressure-vasomotor oscillation. But other non-linear effects also occur, like the entrainment of the slow components that are thought to be associated with thermal adjustments of body core temperature mediated by superficial blood flow.

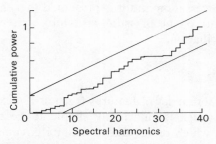

FIG. 3.10. Cumulative normalized a.c. power in harmonics 1–40 of a single 1024-interval sequence. Using the hypothesis of uniform spectral power density, the Kolmogorov–Smirnov critical levels for $P = 0.05$ are shown.

The fluctuations of amplitude and frequency of the pressure-vasomotor component can be studied by complex demodulation, (Sayers 1975*b*). In this procedure, the instantaneous product is formed, throughout the record, of the cardiac interval signal and a complex sinusoid at a reference frequency (a reasonable estimate of the vasomotor frequency is needed); both real and imaginary resultants are then low-pass filtered to 'demodulate' the record. Each original data-point is thus caused to generate a complex number, which is then converted to polar form; the amplitude indicates the relative importance of the component identified at or near the reference frequency, while the curve of phases of the successive complex numbers can be used to indicate actual frequency (in the vicinity of the reference frequency) of the component found. The slope of the phase versus time (sample number) curve is the key to interpretation—a non-zero slope during a part of the record specifies that the operative frequency deviates (proportionately to slope) from the reference frequency, over the appropriate region.

By use of this technique it is possible to establish certain interesting aspects of this component and its interaction: for example, the range of periodicity encompassed by the pressure-vasomotor oscillation (say, 8–12 s), and the changes in frequency that occur near the times when the oscillation evidently stops. Broadly, there are apparently two mechanisms by which this oscillation can be varied and indeed terminated—by entrainment due to respiratory movements of sufficient rate and depth, and by reduction of the apparent time delay which, it is suspected, occurs between the afferent–efferent interface in the brain stem (this can be observed by comparing the latency between pressure-vasomotor component oscillations simultaneously viewed in blood-pressure and in heart-rate). Certainly it is often observed that the oscillatory frequency rises rapidly just prior to cessation and it is presumed that the loop properties (phase shift and gain) of the pressure-vasomotor system are then inadequate to sustain oscillation.

3.4. Pattern analysis

A pattern is a coherent set of features (such as a maximum, minimum, trend, or plateau, which is sufficiently simple to be recognizable as a specific entity, and which recurs under definite circumstances. The only circumstances in which recognizable, and to some extent, reproducible heart-rate patterns are generated is in the response to some stimulation. The onset of physical work load or a change in respiratory pattern, or of a stimulus to the autonomic nervous system, comes into this category, and there is some interest in the possibility of consistent heart-rate responses to mental-load stimuli.

On the other hand, a spontaneous or stimulated pattern change may be restricted to the character of the interval record, rather than producing an explicit waveform. In this case, because of the importance of the phase spectrum in dictating the general form of a pattern, attention would be focused on the phase spectral increments from one harmonic to the next over the relevant band. Existence of a pattern would imply a limited rate of phase increment, and the extent of typical spontaneous fluctuations in this measure needs to be known in order to detect significant alterations.

Coherent averaging of 'stimulated records'

Provided that the stimulus can be repeated so as to allow formation of an ensemble of responses, each with a comparable reference instant, a coherent average—i.e. the ensemble mean—of the post-reference cardiac response, can be formed. The interval signal or perhaps an interpolated interval or rate signal developed from the continuous underlying-signal model discussed above, might be used. (Fig. 3.11 illustrates this approach with the interval variations following the generation of short, standardized speech messages.)

However, there are two difficulties about this kind of ensemble

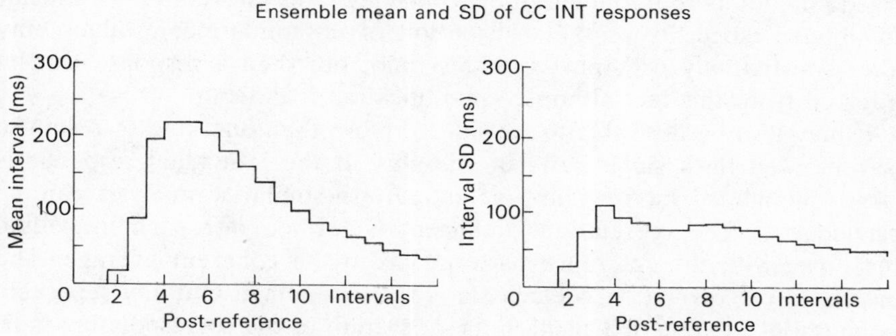

FIG. 3.11. Ensemble average and standard deviation of the pattern of interval magnitude fluctuations due to the production of brief standardized speech messages by the subject (traffic controller). The abscissa is sequential interval number following the start of speaking; the ordinate is interval magnitude increase over the starting value. The ensemble contains 150 such responses.

analysis: the statistical quantification needed to confirm the significance of any results—especially in the ensemble mean (i.e. coherent-average), and the effect of variable latency of pattern features between members of the ensemble.

To identify any explicit features of the response (a peak at time t_1 say, relative to the stimulus) the ensemble mean of the response at t_1 must be shown to be significantly different from that at other times, say t_2. Expressing the difference in ensemble-mean values at these times in relation to the corresponding ensemble standard deviations is often not helpful because the distribution of response values at any post-stimulus time is often far from gaussian. In fact, if repeated stimuli are spaced unsuitably, some of the slow additive oscillatory fluctuations in heart-rate can turn the ensemble distribution of individual values into a bimodal form; this occurs because the periodicities cannot easily be suppressed except by determined effort to utilize a long sequence of random-interval stimuli, which is rarely convenient. The usual small-sample statistical tests are then seriously misleading and there is no basis for converting deviation from the mean into estimated occurrence probability. Further, successive values down the ensemble are then not necessarily independent and the number of degrees of freedom may be much less than the number of members of the ensemble.

Four pieces of information are required for this purpose: the difference in ensemble-mean values, the ensemble standard-deviation, the nature of the distribution of ensemble-mean values, and the number of degrees of freedom contained in the ensemble of values. This information is difficult to obtain, especially as the distribution of ensemble-mean values may alter substantially with post-stimulus time; but then a response can be inferred from this fact although quantification is difficult.

It may also be desirable to consider if more than one kind of response is generated by a single kind of stimulus. If the individual response is large enough to be recognizable, a pattern-similarity analysis can be carried out. The correlation coefficient is formed, for each individual response, with the reference pattern due to the coherent average. The ensemble of correlation coefficients is then examined and any separable populations identified. This permits separation of the corresponding individual responses according to their general form and if, as commonly occurs, there are several different response-patterns, their separate coherent average will provide an estimate of the patterns. The technique has been described in detail in a different field by Sayers and Mansourian (1977).

Feature analysis

If a number of features can be recognized in a stimulated record, then even if variable latency prevents the effective use of coherent averaging, an average response profile may still be determinable. The procedure depends upon the the identification (preferably by some objective method) of the individual features in the individual record, followed by a determination of the magnitude and (timing) location of each. A histogram of each is then compiled from the ensemble of responses and a suitable statistical property (mean, mode, median) selected for each. Thus a series of points are specified, in magnitude and location, which can be linked up to represent a complete average profile of responses: the more features included, the less rudimentary the average profile that results.

The effectiveness of this approach depends on the determination of the individual features, which may perhaps be located visually, or if the response continues for a sufficient number of post-stimulus points (e.g. intervals) by an objective method based on trend analysis. The individual response is processed by the Brown-Trigg procedure (see above) from which the instants at which trends in the response start, finish, or change sign are detected with adequate statistical confidence. In view of the required start-up length of the method, it may be necessary to apply the trend analysis from the end of the post-stimulus record backwards towards the start. Otherwise the detection of early rapid changes may be confused by the start-up responses of the trend filter (Thai Thien Nghia 1977).

3.5. Conclusion

There are three major issues that bear on the cardiac interval (heart-rate) signal and its analysis. First, overriding the detailed fluctuations of this variable, and its global description as well as its pattern characterization, is the existence of substantial and somewhat unpredictable non-stationarities. Postural changes, mechanical effort, sensory disturbances, and spontaneous physiological adjustments are identifiable factors that certainly contribute, but it is not possible to account for much of either transient or sustained non-stationarity. The record must be segmented, and if necessary recompiled into effectively stationary classes, before a valid and complete account of its properties can be obtained in global and detailed terms.

Second, there is very substantial redundancy in the interval record. This is related to characteristics of the interval signal spectrum, from which estimates of $0 \cdot 1 – 0 \cdot 2$ DF per point can be deduced on the basis of a filtered random white Gaussian noise model of the interval signal with only statistical sampling fluctuations. This is broadly consistent with the relation between interval standard deviation and standard error of the mean interval for stationary lengths of record, and despite the questionable applicability of the Gaussian model, is also consistent with the variability of the power in individual components of the interval spectrum (χ^2 with 2 DF, and CV = 1), and of total signal power.

Third, the redundancy can be partly attributed to the presence of several consistent, partially-separable, components in the interval spectrum. There is strong supporting evidence for the proposition that identifiable physiological mechanisms are responsible for these components and the patterns they contribute to the overall fluctuations of the interval sequence. Respiratory and related activity, arterial pressure regulation, and thermally-relevant adjustments of superficial blood flow, are thought to be involved, and since these systems can individually respond to different physiological demands and disturbances, it is certainly useful to separate the signal into components as far as possible before detailed further analysis or, of course, before studying the individual systems. Both linear (e.g. band-selective filtering) and non-linear (e.g. complex modulation) procedures are useful for this purpose.

The presence of effects contributed by dynamic physiological systems is thus one reason why discernible patterns emerge in the interval sequence. Another potential cause is the presence of physical or physiological disturbances, or of autonomically-mediated sensory effects; if interest is to be focused on such factors, the spontaneous fluctuations must again be taken into account. Particularly in such circumstances, if the patterns are recurrent and stable, they may be quantifiable using a coherent-average approach even if the pattern features are small in relation to the background. If the disturbances in question are under the experimenter's control, then varying the interval between successive repetitions may help to maximally suppress the spontaneous background. When the patterns are not stable, then a feature analysis approach would be more appropriate to abstract the general properties of the feature locations and magnitudes, and form an average profile of the pattern. If the patterns merely comprise a general influence on the character of the interval sequence, then spectral descriptions might suffice, provided that the phase spectrum (taking into account its complexities due to delay effects and 'wrap-around' due to principal-angle limits) is also considered.

At the other end of the time-scale, the long-term behaviour of the cardiac interval signal is affected more notably by the irregular appearance of slow non-stationarities of unknown origin. In a complete account of the signal, the nature of these non-stationarities (which signal and statistical parameters are affected?) and the statistics of their occurrences, must be considered and explained. This remains a task for, *inter alia*, ambulatory monitoring.

Acknowledgement

This work has been supported by the Medical Research Council.

References

BENDAT, J. S. and PIERSOL, A. G. (1966). *Measurement and analysis of random data*. Wiley, New York.

BLACKMAN, R. B. and TUKEY, J. W. (1958). The measurement of power spectra. Dover, New York.

BROWN, R. G. (1962). *Smoothing, forecasting, and prediction of discrete time series*. Prentice-Hall, Englewood Cliffs, New Jersey.

COX, D. R. and LEWIS, P. A. (1966). *The statistical analysis of series of events*. Methuen, London.

HYNDMAN, B. W. (1974). The role of rhythms in homeostasis. *Kybernetik* **15**, 227–36.

——, KITNEY, R. I., and SAYERS, B. McA. (1971). Spontaneous rhythms in physiological control systems. *Nature* **233**, 339–41.

LEWIS, C. D. (1971). Statistical monitoring techniques. *Med. biol. Engng* **9**, 315–23.

LYNN, P. A. (1977). On-line digital filters for biological signals: some fast designs for a small computer. *Med. biol. Engng Comput.* **15**, 534–40.

MONRO, D. M. (1975). Complex discrete fast Fourier transform. Algorithm AS83. *Appl. Stat.* **24**, 153–60.

—— (1976). Real discrete fast Fourier transform. Algorithm AS97. *Appl. Stat.* **25**, 166–72.

—— (1977). A portable integer FFT in Fortran. *Comput. Prog. Biomed.* **7**, 267–72.

—— and BRANCH J. L. (1977). The Chirp discrete Fourier transform of general length. Algorithm AS117. *Appl. Stat.* **26**, 351–61.

SAYERS, B. McA. (1970). Inferring significance from biological signals. In *Biomedical engineering systems* (eds M. Clynes and J. H. Milsum), pp. 84–164. McGraw-Hill, New York.

—— (1973). Analysis of heart rate variability. *Ergonom.* **16**, 17–32.

—— (1975a). Physiological consequences of information load and overload. In

Research in psychophysiology (eds P. H. Venables and M. J. Christie), pp. 95–124. Wiley, New York.

—— (1975*b*). The analysis of biological signals. In *Medinfo '74: Proceedings of the Medical Informatics Conference, Stockholm 1974* (eds J. M. Forsythe and J. Anderson), pp. 11–25, 1171–9. North-Holland, Amsterdam.

—— and MANSOURIAN, P. G. (1977). Pattern analysis of epidemiological variables applied in the study of weanling diarrhoeal disease. *Med Informatics* **2**, 69–81.

——, BEAGLEY, H. A., and RIHA, J. (1979). Pattern analysis of auditory-evoked EEG potentials. *Audiology* **18**, 1–16.

SIEGEL, S. (1956). *Non-parametric statistics for the behavioural sciences.* McGraw Hill, New York.

THAI THIEN NGHIA, M. (1977). The implementation and use of statistical signal trend analysis for clinical and epidemiological data. Ph.D. Thesis, Engineering in Medicine Laboratory, Imperial College, University of London.

TRIGG, D. W. (1964). Monitoring a forecasting system. *Operational Res. Quart.* **15**, 271–74.

4.
The assessment of fluctuations in heart-rate
O. ROMPELMAN

4.1. Introduction

THE human heart-rate, even in the normal resting subject, displays continuous fluctuations. In this chapter we will discuss the problem of generating a heart-rate variability (HRV) signal, some hypotheses relating to the underlying mechanisms of different HRV components, and finally a number of different signal analysis methods and their applicability in the study of the aforementioned mechanisms. The material to follow draws upon other work (viz. Rompelman, Coenen, and Kitney 1977).

4.2. HRV signals

The heart-rate can be defined as the rate of occurrence of the cardiac beats, usually expressed in beats per minute. The heart-rate information is often derived from the ECG. The first step in doing so is to reduce the ECG to an event process, the events being the R waves or sometimes the P waves. The second step is to calculate the rate of occurrence of the derived events. In clinical applications the heart-rate is normally identical to the ventricular rhythm, which means that it is derived from the R waves. When relating the heart-rate to the neural cardio-vascular system, the firing rate of the sino-atrial (SA) node is the parameter of interest.

This rate should be derived from the onsets of the P waves in the ECG. In practice however the series of R wave reference moments is used since it is much easier to detect R waves with sufficient accuracy (e.g. 5 ms). It is assumed then, however, that the PR interval is relatively constant i.e. the fluctuations in the PR interval are small in comparison to the detection inaccuracies. In the cardiological field it is generally accepted that under normal circumstances the PR interval is constant; the accuracy limits however are not usually given (e.g. Chung 1971). An analysis of the differences between PP intervals and RR intervals showed that the mean value of these differences was zero with a variance of 3 ms. These values were obtained with ECGs of resting subjects, sampled at a frequency of 1000 Hz. An analysis of some exercise ECGs showed comparable results, viz. zero mean value and a slightly increased variance of 5 ms (de Kok 1975).

It may therefore be concluded that the R wave is indeed a fiducial marker for the SA node activity when the fixed time delay is taken into account.

Turning to heart-rate variability, this variable can be defined as the quantified fluctuations of the heart-rate. These fluctuations are either statistical or deterministic but perturbed by noise. Considering HRV in relation to the neural cardio-vascular system, the fluctuations in general are rather small; large beat-to-beat fluctuations do not occur. The analysis of HRV can be approached in two ways.

First, statistical measures can be employed to describe variability in relation to well defined tasks, as is done in ergonomic physiology. Two examples of these measures are: standard deviation of the RR intervals and the mean value of the absolute differences between two successive heartbeats. This approach is found in later chapters of this monograph. In addition we may refer to the proceedings of the 'Symposium on heart rate variability' which appeared in *Ergonomics* in 1973.

Second, heart-rate variability can be analysed by a signals approach, which implies either the employment of event series analysis methods or the derivation of a signal which is a fair description of the variability. This chapter is devoted to the second approach. Since the fluctuations are small and slow in comparison to the mean heart-rate, this approach is favoured, because it gives a huge data reduction. To give an example: when the R waves are detected with an accuracy of 2 ms, which is not extremely high for event process analysis, a sampling frequency of 500 Hz is needed. The bandwidth of a typical signal describing heart-rate variability might be restricted to, say, 0·5 Hz, yielding a minimum sampling frequency of 1 Hz. This means a data reduction by a factor of 500. Deriving a signal from the R-wave event series can be done in several ways. Four of the more commonly used methods will now be discussed.

In Fig. 4.1, the first two methods are shown. Referring to Fig. 4.1 it can be seen that variations in the RR interval are expressed in two ways. On top we see the ECG, below the derived R wave process. On the left the interval tachogram is shown; here the RR intervals T_1, T_2, etc. are plotted as a function of the interval number. This plot can be considered as a regularly sampled waveform. However, since this plot is a function of the interval number rather than time, care should be taken when this

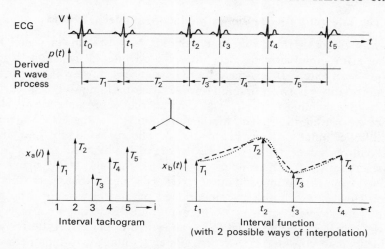

FIG. 4.1. Generation of the interval tachogram and the (interpolated) interval function.

signal is processed for further analysis. For instance a Fourier transform of this signal will not, in fact, yield ordinary frequencies: the units of the abscissa are cycles per interval rather than Hz. An advantage of this method is its simplicity. This method was used by Sayers (1973). It is also discussed in Chapter 3. On the right of Fig. 4.1, a slightly different plot is shown, the so-called interval function. Here the RR intervals are plotted as a function of time. The generated function only differs from zero at the event occurrence times, the value of the function always being the time interval between that particular event and its preceding event. This plot can be considered as an irregularly sampled waveform, which is a time signal unlike the tachogram. By means of interpolation one can obtain a continuous signal which can be sampled regularly for digital processing. This method was used, for example, by Luczak and Laurig (1973).

A third signal is the so-called instantaneous heart-rate, which is in fact the series of reciprocals of RR intervals plotted as a function of time. An application of this method is described by Womack (1971).

A fourth method was indicated by Hyndman and Mohn (1973) and is discussed also in Chapter 10. Here by means of a sharp cut-off, low-pass filter the event series was converted to a slowly varying signal which is representative for heart-rate variability. This signal was called the low-pass filtered event series (LPFES).

61

4.3. The integral pulse frequency modulator model (IPFM)

Having discussed four different methods for obtaining a signal that reflects HRV (interval sequence, interpolated interval function, instantaneous heart-rate, and low-pass filtered event series), we will now discuss the interrelations between them. However, before doing so it is important to note that defining a specific signal as a 'true' representation of HRV implies two assumptions. The first assumption is that the total vagal and sympathetic influence on heart-rate is encompassed in one time-dependant variable $x(t)$; $x(t)$ causes a sort of modulation of the cardiac event series $p(t)$. The second assumption is, that the HRV signal $\hat{x}(t)$ obtained from $p(t)$, is an estimate for $x(t)$. This means that we postulate a model which converts the aforementioned parameter $x(t)$ into the fluctuating cardiac event series $p(t)$, whereupon the HRV meter converts $p(t)$ into the signal $\hat{x}(t)$ being equal to (or an estimate for) $x(t)$. Intuitively we are inclined to consider $x(t)$ as the global resultant of sympathetic and parasympathetic effects on the SA node. It should be emphasized however that the definition of an HRV signal only implies a theoretical model and not necessarily a physiological parameter. On the other hand a model with some physiological relevance is of course more preferable than a model without any such relevance. We will come back to this later.

Hyndman and Mohn (1973) came to their low-pass filtering method by employing a so-called IPFM (integral pulse frequency modulator) as a model. The IPFM model is shown in Fig. 4.3. The input signal $m(t)$ is integrated, yielding $y(t)$. When $y(t)$ reaches a fixed reference value R, a pulse is emitted and the integrator is reset to zero. An example of the modulation of the pulse-rate is given: when, for instance, $m(t)$ increases, the pulse-rate increases as well. Bayly (1968) showed that $m(t)$ can be perfectly reconstituted by low-pass filtering the event series. The low-pass filtering method is therefore based on this IPFM model. In Fig. 4.4 the

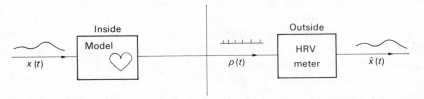

Fig. 4.2. The choice of a particular HRV meter, which converts the cardiac event series $p(t)$ into an HRV signal $\hat{x}(t)$, implies a model, which converts the hypothetical signal $x(t)$ into the cardiac event series $p(t)$, such that $\hat{x}(t) = x(t)$.

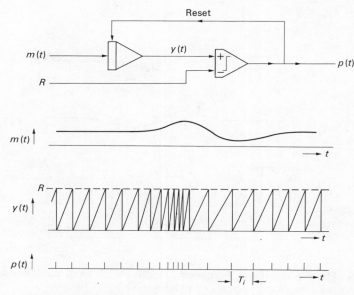

FIG. 4.3. The Integral Pulse Frequency Modulator (IPFM); modulating signal applied to the integrator input; (T_i: pulse interval).

same modulator is shown, but now the input signal is applied to the comparator, whereas the integrator input is kept constant. Again an example of the modulated pulse series is shown.

We now refer to the second method of R wave event series analysis, namely the interval function. Referring to Fig. 4.4, it can be seen that the interpolated interval function of Fig. 4.1 is generated by starting with the event process at the bottom and ending up with the modulating signal $r(t)$. In other words, the application of the interpolated interval function again implies the IPFM model but now the input signal is assumed to be applied to the comparator input.

As pointed out previously, the tachogram is not a function of time. However, if the tachogram is considered as a function of time, then the assumption is that there is a fixed relation between interval number and time. It can be shown that the IPFM model holds in this case as well, provided a non-linear element is inserted between the input, r, and the integrator. This non-linearity appears to have an exponential transfer characteristic. (This is a drawback of the method.)

Finally, the instantaneous heart-rate. It can be shown that the IPFM

63

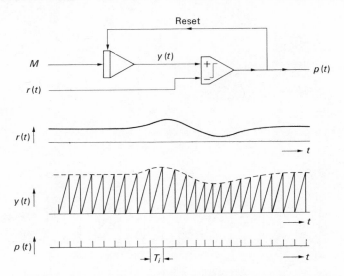

FIG. 4.4. The Integral Pulse Frequency Modulator (IPFM); modulating signal applied to the comparator input; (T_i: pulse interval).

model can be employed as well, provided a non-linear element is inserted in the pathway between the input, m, and the integrator (Rompelman *et al.* 1977). Having discussed the generation of four HRV signals and their relation to the IPFM model, the question arises as to which signal is preferable. Before answering this question, we will state some objectives that should be met:

(1) The model employed should be as simple as possible;
(2) When the HRV signal is fed into the appropriate input of a realization of the model, the output pulse series should be as near as possible to the original cardiac event series even when small errors might have occurred;
(3) The model should have as much physiological relevance as possible.

On the basis of these objectives the interval tachogram is rejected by objective (1) because of the non-linearity involved. The interval function and the instantaneous heart-rate are rejected by objective (2) since small errors in the generation of these signals cause changes in the time events where the signal $y(t)$ crosses the reference value which will cause great differences between the generated and the original event series.

The low-pass filtered event series is based on a simple model.

64

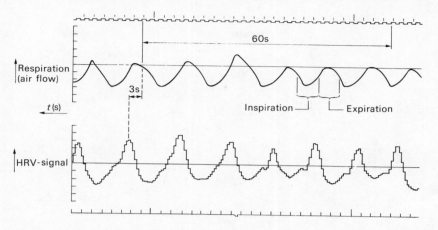

FIG. 4.5. Example of an HRV signal obtained with the hardware filter; for comparison a respiration signal was simultaneously recorded (with a pneumotachograph). (Note the time delay caused by the filter.)

Moreover this model is closest to physiology of all four (as shown, for example, by the results of West, Falk, and Cervioni 1956). Finally, this model is insensitive to small parameter fluctuations when viewed in the light of objective (2) because of the integrator. The conclusion therefore is that the low-pass filtered event series is the most suitable signal for describing heart-rate variability, when studying this phenomenon in relation to the neural cardio-vascular system.

Because of the large data reduction which can be achieved by generating the HRV signal from the ECG, a hardware digital filter for this purpose has been designed (Coenen, Rompelman, and Kitney 1977). This filter has a $\cos^2$ spectral shape. An example of an HRV signal obtained with this filter is shown in Fig. 4.5. The subject showed pronounced respiratory arrhythmia. (Note the inherent frequency-independent time delay between respiration signal and HRV which is due to the symmetrical but time shifted impulse response of the filter.)

4.4. The concept of spontaneous oscillating control systems applied to heart-rate variability

When an HRV signal obtained with the above-mentioned hardware filter is subjected to spectral analysis, the power spectrum can be like

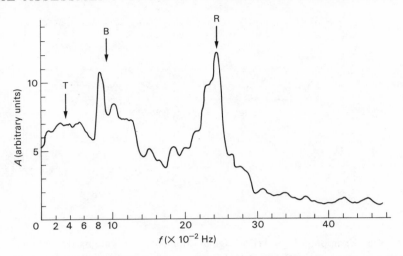

Fɪɢ. 4.6. An example of an HRV spectrum; the three main spectral components are: R, due to respiratory arrhythmia; B, due to blood pressure control system oscillations; and T, due to thermoregulatory control system oscillations.

the example of Fig. 4.6. There are three main spectral regions, indicated by R, B, and T. The peak indicated by R is due to the well-known respiratory arrhythmia and is, of course, located at the respiration frequency. Peak B is usually situated near 0·1 Hz. This peak is considered to be due to an oscillatory character of the blood-pressure control system. Finally, the less pronounced peak T is believed to be caused by the oscillatory character of the thermoregulatory system and is normally in the region around 0·03 Hz. Two of the maxima in the spectrum are thought to be caused by spontaneous oscillations of control systems. Therefore in this section we will give a short introduction to the concept of non-linear control systems and its implications for the analysis of HRV.

Both the blood-pressure and thermoregulatory systems have been subject to thorough investigations. Some authors, however, have indicated that these systems are of a very non-linear character (Sayers 1973). The non-linearity involved can be regarded as a two-sided limiter, or in its idealized form as a so-called 'bang-bang' element. An example of a basic non-linear control system is shown in Fig. 4.7(a). The transfer of the non-linear 'bang-bang' element is shown in Fig. 4.7(b). (The most common realization of such an element is a relay.) It can be shown that the

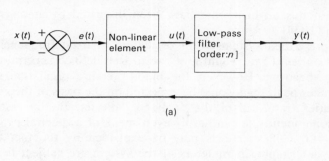

(a)

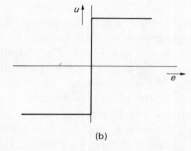

(b)

Fig. 4.7. A basic non-linear control system: (a) block diagram of the system; (b) transfer characteristic of the non-linear 'bang-bang' element.

system is oscillating spontaneously if the phase-lag of the filter exceeds 180° with increasing frequency. Two possible realizations may be a third-order low-pass filter or a pure time delay followed by a low-pass filter of indifferent order. Both amplitude and frequency of the first harmonic of this oscillation can be found analytically by using the describing function method (Gibson 1963). For the reader not familiar with this type of control system, we may refer to the usual domestic heating system. The non-linearity involved is the thermostat, which monitors the difference between its set point and the room temperature. The heater is continuously switched on and off and the actual room temperature displays an oscillation superimposed on the desired mean room temperature.

It has been shown that the thermoregulatory control system is indeed oscillating spontaneously, the frequency of oscillation being about 0·04 Hz (Kitney 1974). This oscillatory behaviour is reflected in HRV as will be discussed in Chapter 5. The blood-pressure control system is also oscillating spontaneously (oscillation frequency about 0·1 Hz) and the influence of this on heart-rate have been discussed by amongst others Hyndman (1974).

If the prescribed systems were oscillating at fixed frequencies their influences on heart rate would give rise to well defined spectral peaks in the HRV spectrum. However, the blood-pressure oscillation shows a much broader peak than would be expected on the basis of the smoothed finite Fourier transform of the analysed data set. In the case of the thermal component one can hardly even speak of a spectral peak (compare Fig. 4.6). These effects may be explained by the fact that the frequency-determining parameters of the system are subject to fluctuations.

The phenomenon of oscillations with fluctuating parameters, which will be referred to as non-stationary oscillations, can be elucidated with the help of the basic system shown in Fig. 4.7. The output signal $y(t)$ displays a natural oscillation under the aforementioned conditions, the frequency of oscillation being f_0. We now assume that one of the frequency-determining parameters of the system is disturbed by an external signal $n_f(t)$, which means that the oscillation frequency f_0 of the system is not constant but fluctuating between f_1 and f_h. (The upper limit of the power spectrum of $n_f(t)$ is assumed to be much less than f_1.) The power spectrum of the output signal $y(t)$ of the oscillatory system then shows a rather broad peak around f_0. (The shape of this peak is related to the probability density function of the amplitude of $n_f(t)$.) Not only the frequency (or the phase) but also the amplitude of the oscillation may be subject to fluctuations, their origin being assumed to be a disturbing signal $n_a(t)$. In order to obtain more information about the disturbing signals $n_f(t)$ and $n_a(t)$ it is necessary to use one of the signal analysis methods to be discussed later.

There are three aspects of interest when applying the concept of non-linear oscillating control systems to different HRV components:

(1) oscillations with unstable amplitude, phase, or frequency;
(2) the phenomenon of frequency selective entrainment;
(3) the physiological background.

The first aspect is the subject of discussion in this chapter, whereas the other two subjects will be discussed in Chapter 5.

4.5. Signal analysis methods

A thorough discussion of signal analysis methods does not seem to be very useful in this context, since a tremendous amount of literature has been published on this subject (e.g. Bendat and Piersol 1971). We will confine ourselves to a short (and incomplete) survey of methods and their possible applications in HRV analysis, keeping in mind that we are interested in the assessment of oscillations and their stability. First we will review some frequency-domain analysis methods and secondly some time-domain analysis methods will be discussed.

Frequency-domain analysis methods

Frequency-domain analysis methods are those methods the results of which are represented as a function of frequency. In Table 4.1 a survey of these methods is given. Since all frequency domain methods involve a time integration viz. the Fourier transform, at first sight they seem to be unsuited for the assessment of non-stationarities. However it is possible to produce so-called running spectra. There are different ways of obtaining running spectra. They are generally based on the principle of repeatedly computing the spectrum of a windowed part of the signal while this part is slowly shifted over the data. In this way one obtains a series of spectra thus showing the spectral properties as a function of time. An example of this procedure will be shown when discussing the coherent averaging technique in the next section. An example of the results of the application of the running spectral analysis will be given in Chapter 5.

Time-domain analysis methods

As we have seen, the straightforward application of frequency-domain analysis methods without the use of special techniques such as running spectra is not suited for the investigation of non-stationary oscillations. We will now discuss some time-domain analysis methods some of them being more suited to our purpose.

Time domain methods for our present purposes are methods the results of which are represented as a function of time or, sometimes time shift. This does not mean that no use is made of frequency-domain data manipulation, as we will see later. In Table 4.2 a survey of time-domain analysis methods is given: the methods indicated will be briefly discussed.

The linear filter can be used in pilot studies. A band filter with a centre frequency corresponding to the frequency of the oscillation under investigation will give a more or less qualitiative impression of the behaviour of that oscillation. The matched filter can be used when predescribed oscillatory patterns (bursts) are to be detected.

Since the auto-correlation function (ACF) and the cross-correlation

TABLE 4.1

A survey of frequency-domain analysis methods applicable in HRV analysis where y(t) is the HRV signal and x(t) is a possible stimulus signal

---

Frequency-domain analysis methods

Basis: the fourier transform (FT)

$$Z(f) = \int_{-\infty}^{+\infty} z(t) e^{-2j\pi ft} \, dt$$

I Power spectrum $Y(f)$
obtained via:
FT of the ACF (Table 4.2)   assessment of oscillations
FFT of the signal, then smoothing   estimate of modulus of frequency
                                         response $H(f)$ of a linear system
                                         by

$$|H(f)|^2 = \frac{Y(f)}{X(f)}$$

II Cross-spectral density $G_{xy}(f) = |G_{xy}(f)| \exp[\varphi_{xy}(f)]$
obtained via:
FT of the CCF (Table 4.2)   estimate of the frequency response
                                 $H(f)$ of a linear system by

$$H(f) = \frac{G_{xy}(f)}{X(f)}$$

time delay τ of a linear system
as a function of frequency by

$$\tau(f) = \frac{\varphi_{xy}(f)}{2\pi f}$$

III Coherence function $\gamma_{xy}^2(f) = \dfrac{G_{xy}(f)^2}{X(f)Y(f)} \leqslant 1$

For a constant linear parameter system: $\gamma = 1$
If $\gamma < 1$, either one or both of the following situations:
extraneous signals present, not correlated with input signal $x(t)$
system relating $x(t)$ and $y(t)$ is not linear

---

function (CCF) are based on time integration, these methods do not seem to be suited for the analysis of non-stationarities. Under certain circumstances, however, it is possible to use a modified correlation technique called the exponentially averaged correlation function. The method is based on the running computation of the correlation function. However, the final function (total) is not a simple average of all calculated functions

TABLE 4.2

A survey of time-domain analysis methods applicable in HRV analysis

Method	Feature
I Linear filter	Separation of desired and undesired signal components
II Matched filter	Detection of known patterns when the occurrence times are not known
III Coherent averaging	Detection of unknown patterns when the occurrence times are known
IV Auto-correlation function	Determination of the degree of randomness
V Cross-correlation function	Determination of phase shift (or time delay)
VI Complex demodulation	Tracking of phase or frequency of non-stationary oscillations
VII Homomorphic filtering	Tracking of amplitude of non-stationary oscillations

but is permanently updated exponentially according to the relation:

New running total = Old running total −

$$- \frac{\text{New calculated function} - \text{Old running total}}{k}$$

in which k is a factor effecting the equivalent time constant of the averaging procedure. This method is applied in the Hewlett and Packard Correlator (type 3721A) (Anderson and Perry 1969).

The coherent averaging technique is a well known method in enhancing the response to a stimulus when this response is buried in noise. This method is also not necessarily restricted to stationary systems. It is possible to carry out a so-called running average (Fig. 4.8). The average response is obtained from n successive sweeps. This window of n stimulus periods is shifted over the process period by period. It can be seen from the figure that both power and phase of the first harmonics of the averaged response are calculated, in each case yielding different time dependent variables describing the non-stationarity of the transfer. This method was used by Kitney and Rompelman (1977) in the analysis of the human thermoregulatory system in relation to HRV; it will also be discussed in Chapter 5.

Complex demodulation and homomorphic filtering are methods most suited to the investigation of unstable oscillations. The procedure of

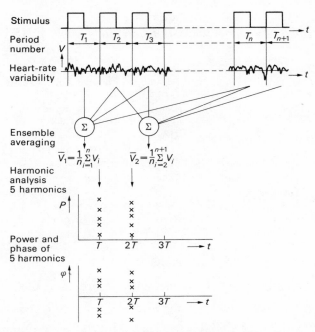

FIG. 4.8. Procedure for computing power and phase of harmonics of a stimulus frequency present in a heart-rate variability signal, and plotted as a function of time.

complex demodulation consists of three main steps. First, the spectral region of interest is shifted to zero frequency, second, the result is low-pass filtered so that only frequency components around zero remain, and, finally, since the result is a complex signal, both amplitude and phase are calculated from this result and plotted as a function of time. A block diagram of a time-domain computation of the complex demodulate is shown in Fig. 4.9. In Fig. 4.10 three examples of theoretical results of complex demodulation are shown when the original signal $y(t) = A \cos(2\pi ft + \gamma)$ is subject to three different types of disturbances. The results can be easily verified. In practice it can be advantageous to do the complex demodulation via the Fourier transform (FFT), frequency-domain filtering, shifting, and inverse Fourier transforming (Fig. 4.11). (Note that the two-sided Fourier transform must be applied.) In Fig. 4.11 two possible filtering windows are shown. The ideal rectangular window (drawn curve) has a main disadvantage being a severe time leakage, which

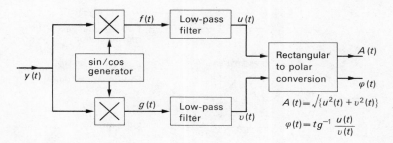

FIG. 4.9. Block diagram of the time domain procedure of complex demodulation.

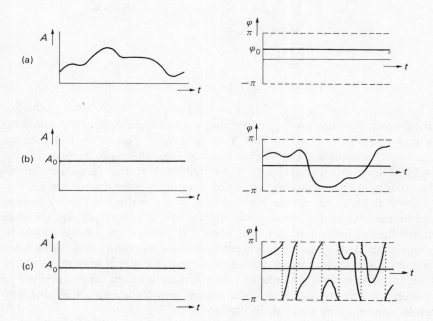

FIG. 4.10. Three theoretical phase results of complex demodulation if the signal to investigate contains a main component $y(t) = \cos(2\pi ft + \gamma)$: (a) unstable amplitude, stable frequency, $A = A(t)$, $f = f_0$, $\gamma = \gamma_0$; (b) stable amplitude, unstable phase, $A = A_0$, $f = f_0$, $\gamma = \gamma(t)$; (c) stable amplitude, unstable frequency, $A = A_0$, $f = f(t)$.

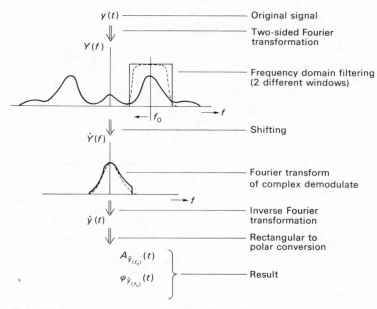

FIG. 4.11. Frequency domain procedure of complex demodulation.

means that transients will penetrate into both the preceding and following signal (Bingham, Godfry, and Tuckey 1967). This drawback can be avoided by applying a smoother window, viz. the dashed curve in Fig. 4.11. However, it can easily be noted that if the frequency of an oscillation is fluctuating in the region around f_f these frequency fluctuations will yield amplitude fluctuations at the output; in other words, frequency fluctuations will penetrate in the amplitude of the complex demodulate. This phenomenon is known as 'slope detection'. It should be emphasized that slope detection also occurs when complex demodulation is carried out in the time domain as described earlier. It may therefore be concluded that complex demodulation is mainly suited for the analysis of fluctuations in frequency when studying non-stationary oscillating systems.

In a preliminary investigation a hybrid computer simulation for interactive complex demodulation was developed. By using this set-up with an HRV signal that showed a double peak near $0\cdot1$ Hz, it was found that this double peak was most likely to be due to one fluctuating frequency rather than two different frequencies (de Vries 1976).

74

Finally, we will briefly discuss a technique introduced by Oppenheim, Schafer, and Stockham (1968) called homomorphic filtering. This technique can be described as a method for separating signals that are related by multiplication rather than addition. (An example may be an oscillation with a fluctuating mean amplitude.)

Assume that a signal $x(t)$ is composed of two components, namely a desired component $s(t)$ and an undesired component $n(t)$ such that $x(t) = s(t) \cdot n(t)$. Homomorphic filtering consists of the three following steps:

(1) Take the logarithm of $x(t)$ yielding $\hat{x}(t) = \hat{s}(t) + \hat{n}(t)$ in which $\hat{s}(t) = \log\{s(t)\}$ and $\hat{n}(t) = \log\{n(t)\}$.
(2) Since $\hat{s}(t)$ and $\hat{n}(t)$ are now related linearly, it is possible to remove $\hat{n}(t)$ by means of a linear filter, resulting in $\hat{s}(t)$.
(3) Take the inverse logarithm of the result $\hat{s}(t)$ of the linear filtering operation yielding the desired signal $s(t)$.

Having discussed the principle, three important points must be made:

(1) Since the logarithm is a very non-linear operation giving rise to a great number of harmonics, a sufficient separation in step (2) can only be obtained if the spectra of $s(t)$ and $n(t)$ are widely divergent.
(2) The appearance of harmonics as a matter of course implies a much higher sampling rate as were needed on the basis of the original signal bandwidth.
(3) Since $x(t)$ is normally a bipolar signal, the introduction of the complex logarithm is needed.

For a thorough treatment of homomorphic filtering we refer to Oppenheim and Schafer (1975).

In conclusion, therefore, it can be said that oscillations with unstable phase or frequency can be analysed by means of complex demodulation, whereas for the analysis of oscillations with a fluctuating amplitude the homomorphic filtering method is more promising. It is important to note, and this holds for frequency- and time-domain methods alike, that the shorter the data set on which the analysis is carried out, the less reliable the results will be. In statistical terms: the confidence intervals of the estimated parameters will increase as the size of the considered data set decreases. This statement is extremely important when analysing non-stationarities.

As discussed earlier, the oscillatory phenomena stem from very non-linear control systems. An important property of these systems is that the oscillations are superimposed on the mean value of the controlled variable. It is hoped that the study of the character of the oscillations rather than the average effects of some control systems might give information about how the systems are operating. Changes in the oscillatory pattern might indicate disturbances before effects in the controlled variables become apparent, in other words: it is hoped that in the future these methods will help to develop techniques applicable in preventive medicine.

4.6. Conclusion

We have seen that defining an HRV signal as a representation of the fluctuations in heart-rate implies a model. The preference of the IPFM model and the consequent choice of the low-pass filtered cardiac event series as a suitable HRV signal have been discussed. The concept of unstable oscillatory systems underlying some particular HRV components has been introduced as well as appropriate signal analysis methods for the investigation of such systems.

References

ANDERSON, G. C. and PERRY, M. A. (1969). A calibrated real time correlator/averager/probability analyser. *Hewlett-Packard J.* November 1969, 9–15.

BAYLY, E. J. (1968). Spectral analysis of pulse frequency modulation in the nervous system. *IEEE Trans. Bio-med. Engng (Inst. elect. electron. Engrs)* **BME-15**, 257–65.

BENDAT, J. S. and PIERSOL, A. G. (1971). *Random data: analysis, measurements, procedures.* Wiley-Interscience, New York.

BINGHAM, C., GODFRY, M. D. and TUCKEY, J. W. (1967). Modern techniques of power spectrum estimation. *IEEE Trans. audio- electro-acoust. (Inst. elect. electron. Engrs)* **AU-15**, 56–66.

CHUNG, E. K. (1971). *Principles of cardiac arrhythmias.* Williams and Wilkins, Baltimore, Maryland.

COENEN, A. J. R. M., ROMPELMAN, O., and KITNEY, R. I. (1977). Measurement of heart rate variability; Part II: Hardware digital device for the assessment of heart rate variability. *Med. biol. Engng Com.* **15**, 423–30.

ERGONOMICS (1973). Proceedings of the Symposium on Heart-rate Variability. *Ergonomics* **16** (1).

GIBSON, J. E. (1963). *Non linear automatic control.* McGraw-Hill, New York.

HYNDMAN, B. W. (1974). The role of rhythms in homeostasis. *Kybernetik* **15**, 227–36.

—— and MOHN, R. K. (1973). A pulse modulator model for pacemaker activity. *Digest of the Xth Intern. Conf. on Med. and Biol. Engng.*, p. 223. Dresden.

KITNEY, R. I. (1974). The analysis and simulation of the human thermoregulatory control system *Med. biol. Engng* **12**, 57–64.

—— and ROMPELMAN, O. (1977). Analysis of the interaction of the human bloodpressure and thermal control systems. In *Biomedical computing* (ed. W. J. Perkins). Pitman Medical, Tunbridge Wells, Kent.

DE KOK, L. A. (1975). *Een onderzoek naar de eventuele aanwezigheid van deterministische komponenten in de slag op slag variaties in de intervaltijden tussen P-golf begin en QRS-komplex.* Delft University of Technology, Biomed. Eng. Group, Internal Report M142.

LUCZAK, H. and LAURIG, W. (1973). An analysis of heart rate variability *Ergonomics*, **16** (1), 85–97.

OPPENHEIM, A. V., SCHAFER, R. W., and STOCKHAM, T. G. (1968). Non linear filtering of multiplied and convolved signals *Proc. IEEE* **56** (8), 1264–91.

—— —— (1975). *Digital signal processing.* Prentice-Hall, Englewood Cliffs, New Jersey.

ROMPELMAN, O., COENEN, A. J. R. M., and KITNEY, R. I. (1977). Measurement of heart rate variability; Part I: Comparative study of heart rate variability analysis methods *Med. biol. Engng Comp.* **17**, 233–9.

SAYERS, B. McA. (1973). Analysis of heart rate variability *Ergonomics* **16** (1), 85–97.

DE VRIES, J. (1976). *Complexe demodulatie.* Delft University of Technology, Biomed. Eng. Group, Internal Report M 151.

WEST, T. C., FALK, G., and CERVIONI, P. (1956). Drug alteration in transmembrane potentials in atrial pacemaker cells *J. Pharmacol. exp. Ther.* **117**, 245–52.

WOMACK, B. F. (1971). The analysis of respiratory simus arrhythmia using spectral analysis methods. *IEEE Trans. Bio-med. Engng* (*Inst. elect. electron. Engrs*), **BME-18** 162, 399–409.

Part III

Applications of heart-rate variability analysis with respect to physiology

5.

An analysis of the thermoregulatory influences on heart-rate variability

R. I. KITNEY

5.1. Introduction

THERMOREGULATION in humans can be roughly divided into three forms of response: shivering, sweating, and vasomotor activity; it is the vasomotor activity which is of interest here. Thermal vasomotor activity can be considered as a fine control mechanism in the regulation of body temperature. In the late-1930s and early-1940s a number of workers (e.g. Burton and Taylor 1940) identified fluctuations in digit blood-flow which they associated with thermal vasomotor activity in the approximate range of 15- to 30-s periodicity.

These oscillations in digit blood-flow formed the basis of our analysis of the nature of the thermal vasomotor control system. The question which was asked was: what kind of control system could produce this type of oscillation? After a careful study of the data, the conclusion which was reached was that the control system must be of the non-linear oscillatory type, i.e. the type of bounded oscillations which were observed must emanate from a non-linear rather than a linear control system. A model of the system will be described later in the text.

In 1962 Minorsky discussed the theory of non-linear oscillatory systems in considerable detail. At this stage in the research it was important to test our deductions relating to the nature of the control system and to this end the property of such systems which Minorsky calls entrainment was extremely important. Minorsky's theory of entrainment formed the basis of a set of experiments (Kitney 1975). The purpose of these was to test the non-linear nature of the thermal vasomotor control system by attempting to entrain the thermal oscillations in digit blood-flow with a periodic thermal stimulus. After a careful study of the physiological literature it was decided that the stimulus should be achieved by placing one hand alternately in two tanks containing water at different temperatures. (In the first set of experiments the temperatures were 18 and 46 °C.)

Consider the case of an experiment in which a 20-s stimulus was applied. In the experiment the subject was asked to place one hand in the cold tank for 10 s followed by 10 s in the warm tank, followed by 10 s in the cold tank, and so on. Variation in finger blood volume were recorded from a photoplethysmogram placed on the small finger of the opposite hand, and the ECG (single chest lead) was recorded on an FM instrumentation tape-recorder for the duration of the experiment (15 min).

In general, for different stimulus frequencies the digit blood-flow in the opposite hand had a dominant frequency component at the stimulus frequency, indicating entrainment. The range of entrainment was found to be about 8 to 80 s (Kitney 1975). Further experiments led to a detailed analysis of the thermal vasomotor control system. The next stage in the research was to study the effect of these thermal stimuli on heart-rate.

Work in the Engineering in Medicine Laboratory at Imperial College led to two papers: Hyndman, Kitney, and Sayers (1971) on the nature of spontaneous rhythms in physiological control systems, and Sayers (1973) on the analysis of heart-rate variability specifically. The essence of these papers as far as heart-rate variability is concerned can be summed up in two statements:

(1) There appear to be three frequency components in the normal heart-rate variability power spectrum which arise from the activity of physiological control systems: a temperature component in the range 0·05 Hz, a blood pressure component at around 0·1 Hz, and a respiratory component at about 0·25 Hz, depending on the respiration rate. (These components can be observed during spontaneous resting conditions.)

(2) These three components arise from the non-linear oscillatory nature of the thermoregulatory, blood-pressure, and respiratory control systems.

The question of interest was therefore whether or not heart-rate could be entrained in a similar manner to blood-flow. If thermal entrainment of heart-rate were possible then this would provide conclusive evidence of the existence of the thermal component in the RR interval power spectrum. Unfortunately, such analysis relies on the RR interval spectrum being expressed in terms of true frequency rather than in beats per interval which is the abscissa scale which results from Fourier transformation of the interval tachogram. The raw RR interval waveform comprise irregular samples and these must be converted to the low-pass filtered event series (LPFES) prior to spectral analysis. When the ECG signals recorded during the original entrainment experiments were analysed in this way, the power spectra showed evidence of entrainment in the period range 5–12 s. What should be borne in mind at this stage is that the range of entrainment of period 5–12 s is based on a series of experiments in which the two tank temperatures were always 18 and 46 °C. Further work with the entrainment of digit blood-flow showed that the range of entrainment was a function of both stimulus frequency and amplitude. A further series of experiments were therefore undertaken in which both stimulus amplitude and frequency were varied incrementally. The results of these experiments confirmed the existence of entrainment in the thermal component of the RR interval waveform, but they also showed that there are three types of entrainment: stable, metastable, and unstable entrainment. These three types will now be described in relation to Fig. 5.1.

1. *Stable entrainment.* Referring to Fig. 5.1, if an input $x(t) = A \cos(\omega_1 t + \phi_1)$ is applied to the non-linear oscillatory system and the output is $y(t) = B \cos(\omega_2 t + \phi_2)$, then for stable entrainment both the amplitude and phase of the output, i.e. B and ϕ_2, are constant. (The thermal component of the LPFES power spectrum will be stable in both amplitude and frequency, such that $\omega_2 = \omega_1$.)

2. *Metastable entrainment.* During metastable entrainment both the amplitude B and the phase ϕ_2 may vary but the frequency of the thermal component remains locked to the stimulus frequency ($\omega_2 = \omega_1$).

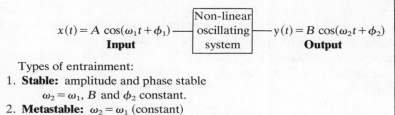

$x(t) = A \cos(\omega_1 t + \phi_1)$ —— Non-linear oscillating system —— $y(t) = B \cos(\omega_2 t + \phi_2)$
Input   **Output**

Types of entrainment:
1. **Stable:** amplitude and phase stable
   $\omega_2 = \omega_1$, B and ϕ_2 constant.
2. **Metastable:** $\omega_2 = \omega_1$ (constant)
   B and ϕ_2 may vary.
3. **Unstable:** ω_2 not always equal to ω_1
   Frequency component sometimes lost,
   B and ϕ_2 very unstable.

FIG. 5.1. The various types of entrainment found in a biological system.

3. *Unstable entrainment.* During unstable entrainment, the output frequency ω_2 is not always equal to the input frequency ω_1, the amplitude and phase of the thermal component of the RR interval waveform (B and ϕ_2) are very unstable and there may be periods when the component at the stimulus frequency (in the LPFES power spectrum) is lost.

5.2. Analysis of the three types of entrainment

As one might expect, the differing properties of the three types of entrainment observed in the thermal component of the LPFES spectrum require different signal analysis techniques. A number of the methods which we have developed or employed have been discussed in Chapter 4. To recapitulate, for stable oscillations the analysis methods are: amplitude and power spectra, measurement of power in the various frequency bands, correlation, averaging, and the coherence function. For unstable oscillations the analysis techniques are: running spectra, running power in the frequency bands, running correlation average, running coherence, and complex demodulation.

The analysis of stable entrainment

As has already been mentioned, the results of the first set of experiments involving the analysis of the HRV waveform defined a range of entrainment having a period between about 5 and 12 s. In order to understand the properties of stable entrainment further, it was decided to look at sets of results which exhibited dominant components at the stimulus frequency where these frequencies were: (a) inside; (b) at the edge of; and (c) outside, the range of entrainment. Consider an example taken from the analysis of three stimulus frequencies which fit these criteria: stimuli with periods of 10, 16, and 20 s, respectively. The important point to note is that the LPFES spectra all showed evidence of stable entrainment and the question was whether or not there were differences.

Analysis of cross-correlation. Cross-correlating the HRV waveforms with sine waves of the same periodicities as the stimuli and also with spontaneous data, showed that there was significantly greater correlation when the sine wave at the stimulus frequency was used. There was some correlation with the spontaneous data, and no correlation in the case of the other sine waves. The coherence function was computed in each case and had values in excess of 0·9 for the high values of correlation.

Power in the frequency bands. In this part of the analysis the spectral power in various frequency bands of the LPFES power spectrum during the application of the stimulus was compared with that obtained from spontaneous data. The results are illustrated in Fig. 5.2(a). Referring to

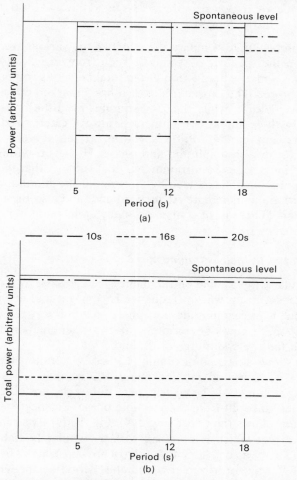

FIG. 5.2. (a) Power in different frequency bands of the LPFES for different stimulus frequencies. (b) Total power in the LPFES for different stiumulus frequencies.

85

Fig. 5.2, for the 10-s stimulus the power in the 5–12-s band was significantly less during the application of the stimulus. There was some reduction in power in the 12–18-s band and no significant reduction in the >18-s band. The 16-s stimulus caused a significant reduction in the 12–18-s band (of the same order as that observed for the 10-s stimulus) and some reduction in the other two bands. The 20-s stimulus resulted in some reduction in power in the >18-s band but had little or no effect on the power in the other bands.

It is also interesting to compare the effect of the various stimuli on the total power in the spectrum. As can be seen from Fig. 5.2(b), the 10-s stimulus causes a marked reduction in the total power as compared to the spontaneous power. The 16-s stimulus also has a marked effect, although not quite as significant, while the 20-s stimulus has little or no effect.

In summary then, stable entrainment is always categorized by a frequency component in the LPFES spectrum at the stimulus frequency which is stable in both amplitude and phase. However, within the type there are varying degrees of entrainment—that is to say that the degree of stable entrainment may be defined by the amount the stimulus can reduce the power within its immediate frequency band, and also the total power in the spectrum. (There is, of course, normally an increase in power at the stimulus frequency.)

The analysis of metastable entrainment

To recapitulate, metastable entrainment is categorized by a component in the LPFES spectrum whose frequency is constant and at the stimulus frequency, but whose amplitude and phase may vary in relation to the stimulus. Fig. 5.3 shows an example of the phenomenon for a 10-s stimulus with tank temperatures of 22 and 37 °C.

The figure shows a 512-point running LPFES spectrum computed from a 256-s data window and moving along 100 samples at a time. The instability in amplitude can be clearly seen. In fact the unstable amplitude normally seems to result from the unstable phase. Perspective plotting of the HRV signal shows the effect (Fig. 5.4). Fig. 5.4(a) illustrates the type of perspective plot which is obtained with a completely stable thermal component. (The plots of Fig. 5.4(a) and (b) are constructed by dividing a length of HRV waveform into two stimulus period segments with time increasing from front to back.) The effect of metastability can clearly be seen by comparing the two figures. In the metastable case (b) both the amplitude and phase of the waveform are varying.

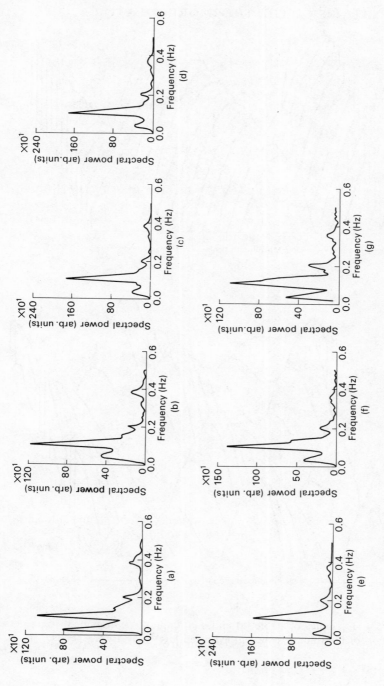

Fig. 5.3. An example of metastable entrainment with a 10-s thermal stimulus.

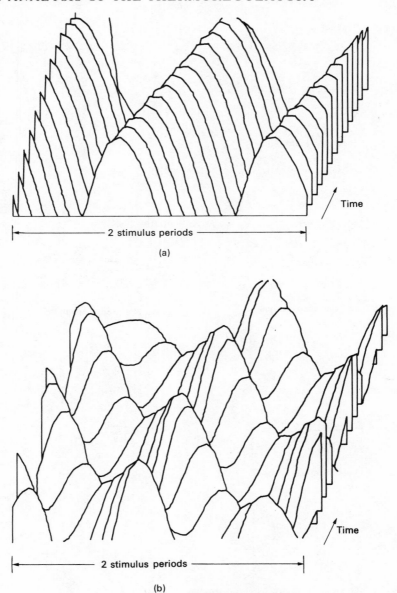

FIG. 5.4. Examples of stable (a) and metastable (b) entrainment using perspective plots of the running coherent averaged HRV waveform (see also Ch. 4).

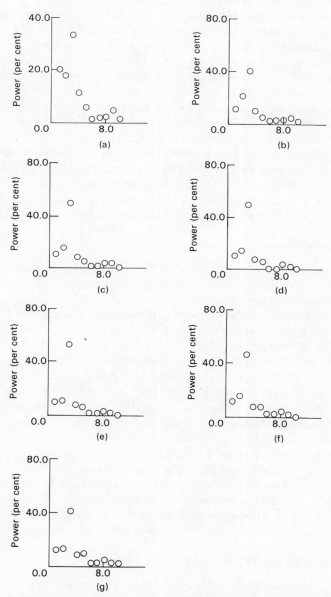

FIG. 5.5. Power distribution in various frequency bands of the LPFES showing a transition from metastable to stable entrainment.

The most effective means of studying the phenomenon of metastability seems to be the running phase spectrum. In this application, the phase of the first harmonic (stimulus frequency) is plotted as a function of time. Stable entrainment produces a flat phase spectrum while for metastability the flat regions are interspersed with areas of unstable phase. (The method is fully discussed in Kitney and Rompelman (1977).

The transition from metastability to full stability can also clearly be seen by computing the power in the bands from the 512-point running LPFES power spectra, as shown in Fig. 5.5.

In summary, therefore, metastable entrainment differs from stable entrainment by virtue of the fact that the amplitude and phase of the stimulus component in the HRV power spectrum varies. Our results indicate that it is the phase which is the important factor, particularly when one is observing the transition from metastability to full stability.

Unstable entrainment

The condition of unstable entrainment is categorized (referring to Fig. 5.1) by a combination of the following conditions:
(1) ω_2 is not always equal to ω_1;
(2) the stimulus frequency component sometimes disappears from the LPFES power spectrum;
(3) B and ϕ_2 are very unstable.

Fig. 5.6 illustrates this phenomenon. Referring to Fig. 5.6(a), even though a thermal stimulus is present throughout the record, there is no evidence of it in the power spectrum. However, if the LPFES waveform is examined more closely, it becomes clear that there are sections of the waveform where there is an oscillation at the stimulus frequency—this is an example of unstable entrainment.

Hence the phenomenon of unstable entrainment occurs in the presence of a constant thermal stimulus. The exact reason why the waveform switches from one state to another at a particular time is often obscure. Nevertheless, unstable entrainment is frequently caused by either bursts of biological noise or non-linear beating between the stimulus and the other physiological oscillations which form the HRV waveform.

5.3. The control theory basis of the mechanism

Fig. 5.7 illustrates the control theory model which has been developed to describe the nature of the physiological oscillations which have been observed (Hyndman *et al.* 1971). Referring to Fig. 5.7, the model is of the

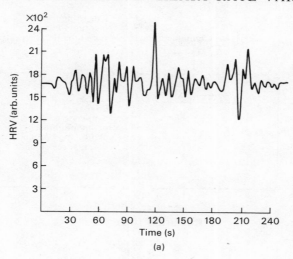

(a)

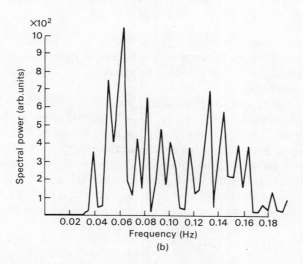

(b)

FIG. 5.6. An example of unstable entrainment (6-s thermal stimulus) where the power spectrum (b) shows no evidence of the stimulus while regions of the LPFES do.

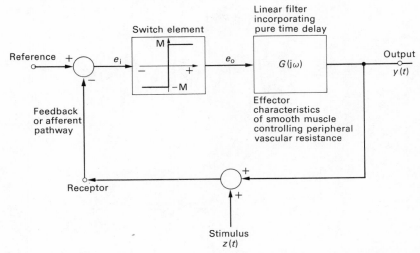

FIG. 5.7. The control theory model which was developed to stimulate physiological oscillations. (See also Chapter 10.)

negative-feedback-type and comprises three basic sections: the linear characteristics of the peripheral vascular bed, a pure time delay, and a non-linear switch element (usually referred to in control theory as a 'bang-bang' element).

The characteristics of the peripheral vascular bed have been studied by a number of workers since Scher and Young (1963). Examples are: Levison, Barnet, and Jackson (1966), Spickler, Kezdi, and Geller (1967), Rosenbaum and Rice (1968). In each case the results were only variations on Scher and Young's original findings. Consequently in the present study we concentrated on Scher and Young's original data. The frequency response $G(j\omega)$ of the peripheral vascular bed was computed from Scher and Young's data by a least squares fitting technique and found to be:

$$G(j\omega) = \frac{22 \cdot 0(1 + 12j\omega)}{(1 + 92j\omega)(1 + 2j\omega)}.\qquad(5.1)$$

Referring to the Nyquist plot shown in Fig. 5.8, it is clear that the locus does not encircle the -1 point, which is the condition for oscillation Kuo (1967). The incorporation of the pure time delay in the model changes this situation dramatically. The amount of time delay required to produce the oscillation frequencies observed physiologically can be derived analytically as follows.

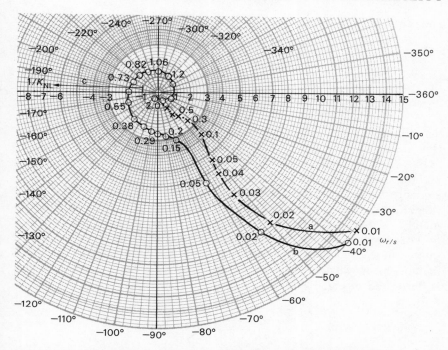

FIG. 5.8. The Nyquist loci of the peripheral vascular resistance: (a) without pure time delay and (b) with a time delay of 3·3 s.

The open loop transfer function of the model including pure time delay is

$$G(j\omega) = \frac{22 \cdot 0 (1 + 12 j\omega) e^{-j\omega T}}{(1 + 92 j\omega)(1 + 2 j\omega)}. \tag{5.1}$$

Rationalizing and removing the gain term (it is irrelevant here),

$$G'(j\omega) = \frac{(1 + 12 j\omega)(1 - 92 j\omega)(1 - 2 j\omega) e^{-j\omega T}}{(1 + (92\omega)^2)(1 + 4\omega^2)}. \tag{5.2}$$

Now, the point of oscillation occurs when the locus crosses the negative real axis of the Nyquist plane. At this point the imaginary part of $G(j\omega)$ is zero.

Expanding the numerator of eqn (5.2),

$$\cos \omega T - j \sin \omega T - 2 j\omega \cos \omega T - 2\omega \sin \omega T - 80 j\omega \cos \omega T$$
$$- 80\omega \sin \omega T - 160\omega^2 \cos \omega T + 160 j\omega^2 \sin \omega T + 1104\omega^2 \cos \omega T$$
$$- 1104 j\omega^2 \sin \omega T - 2208 j\omega^3 \cos \omega T - 2208\omega^2 \sin \omega T$$

93

and, equating the imaginary part to zero,

$$\sin \omega T + 2\omega \cos \omega T + 80\omega \cos \omega T - 160\omega^2 \sin \omega T$$
$$+ 1104\omega^2 \sin \omega T + 2208\omega^2 \cos \omega T = 0$$

or

$$944 \tan(\omega T)\omega^2 + 82\omega + 2208\omega^3 + \tan \omega T = 0. \qquad (5.3)$$

The solution of eqn (5.3) defines the oscillation frequency for a particular time delay T.

Fig. 5.9 illustrates the relationship between the oscillation frequency and the value of the delay. There is a reasonable amount of physiological evidence for such a delay. Scher and Young (1963) quote a delay in the range 2–4·5 s, while Hatakegama (1967) observed a delay of approximately 2 s. Rosenbaum and Rice on the other hand mention a delay but do not specify a value. It is interesting to note that the delays which are quoted in these papers are consistent with the solution of eqn (5.3). The Nyquist locus which results from a time delay of 3·3 s (0·1 Hz oscillation) is illustrated in Fig. 5.8.

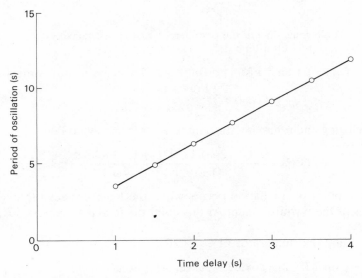

FIG. 5.9. The relationship between the period of the oscillation of the system and the value of the time delay. (Calculated from the model of Fig. 5.7.)

Although the basic conditions for oscillation are satisfied by the linear characteristics and the pure time delay the oscillation will in practice be unstable. When the critical point lies to the left of $G(j\omega)$ locus or is not enclosed by it, the poles of the closed loop transfer function have negative real parts. The system is then stable since any disturbances which appear tend to die out. Conversely, when the critical point lies to the right of the $G(j\omega)$ locus and is therefore enclosed by it, the poles of the closed loop transfer function have positive real parts and the system is unstable. If $G(j\omega)$ passes through the -1 point the system may have a sustained oscillation which is either stable or unstable. If a slight disturbance in amplitude or frequency occurs and the oscillation returns to its original value, the oscillation is stable. Alternatively, if the oscillation continues to increase or decrease it is unstable.

In a physiological system, by virtue of its nature, disturbances will certainly occur. Clearly both an unstable oscillation or a decaying oscillation is inconsistent with the physiological situation. It is therefore necessary to consider what additional element is required to stabilize the oscillation. The non-linear elenent which is appropriate is the bang-bang or switch element. There is some physiological evidence for the existence of such an element. Grodins (1963) discusses its physiological existence and Scher and Young (1963) introduces the sgn function into their analysis. The effect of the element on the behaviour of the model can be readily understood by using the describing function technique (Gibson 1963) in conjunction with the Nyquist plane. Referring to Fig. 5.8 the locus of the bang-bang element in the Nyquist plane lies along the negative real axis and starts at the -1 point. If the equivalent gain of the describing function is K_{NL}, then the condition for a sustained oscillation becomes $K_{NL} G(j\omega) = -1$ or $G(j\omega) = -1/K_{NL}$ and the stable oscillation occurs at the intersection of the two loci. More detailed studies by Hyndman (1970), Kitney (1972, 1975), and Kitney, Rompelman, and Spruyt (1976) have shown that the model is consistent with the experimental results and can be used to study the entrainment phenomenon.

5.4. Analysis of the model by describing function techniques

The model illustrated in Fig. 5.7 can be analysed in greater detail using the describing function technique. The basis of the method is as follows: the non-linearity is treated separately and a new function, the describing function, is derived which defines its behaviour. Referring to Fig. 5.7, it is assumed that the input to the non-linearity $e_i(t)$ is a sine wave (which is true for the self-sustained oscillation) and that $e_i(t) = A \sin \omega t$. The output from the non-linearity will be a periodic function which can be described by a Fourier series of the form:

$$e_0(t) = \sum_{n=1}^{\infty} (a_n \cos n\omega t + b_n \sin n\omega t).$$

(It is assumed that the non-linearity does not give rise to a d.c. term.) The describing function is defined as: $D(A, \omega) =$ the fundamental of $e_0(t)/\text{input}$, $e_i(t)$. If the range of the switch element is $\pm M$, and $e_i(t) = A \sin \omega t$, then

$$e_0(t) = \frac{4M}{\pi} (\sin \omega t + \tfrac{1}{3} \sin 3\omega t + \tfrac{1}{5} \sin 5\omega t)$$

and the describing function $D(A, \omega)$ is

$$D(A, \omega) = \frac{\dfrac{4M}{\pi} \sin \omega t}{A \sin \omega t} = \frac{4M}{\pi}.$$

Therefore the equivalent gain of the non-linearity, $K_{NL} = 4M/\pi A$. The simple describing function approach only works however, when the system is oscillating spontaneously in the absence of an external stimulus. Referring to Fig. 5.7, it is clear that the condition of entrainment occurs because of the presence of such a stimulus. A method which is a more sophisticated version of the describing function technique, the dual input describing function of DIDF) has been developed to cater for this need. Boyer (1960) discusses the way in which the DIDF can be derived for a particular system non-linearity. The method is presented in abbreviated form by Gibson (1963) and is often difficult to follow. Consequently, a modified and, hopefully, clearer version will now be given.

If the external stimulus $z(t)$ has the form $B \cos \omega t$ then the input to the non-linearity $e_i(t)$ becomes

$$e_i(t) = A \sin \omega t + B \cos \beta t.$$

In order to simplify the derivation of the dual input describing function it is assumed that $\beta > \omega$.

The first stage in the derivation is to determine the so-called equivalent d.c. gain of the non-linearity, which is defined as:

$$K(A_0, B) = \frac{\text{average value of the output}}{\text{average value of the input}} = \frac{A_v}{A_0}$$

where the input is given by $e_i(t) = A_0 + B \sin \beta t...$, i.e. the low-frequency component is assumed to be constant.

Hence for a particular value of the low-frequency component of the input A_0 the output waveform will be as shown in Fig. 5.10(b) the input to the non-linearity $e_i(t)$, being

$$e_i(t) = A_0 + B \cos \beta t.$$

Hence the output $e_0(t)$ from the non-linearity will be

$$-M \quad \text{if} \quad e_i(t) < 0$$

and

$$+M \quad \text{if} \quad e_i(t) \geqslant 0$$

and for $|A_0| \leqslant |B|$, $e_0(t)$ will be positive if $B \cos \beta t > -A_0$. Therefore,

$$\cos \beta t > -\frac{A_0}{\beta} \quad \text{and} \quad |\beta t| < \cos^{-1}\left\{\frac{-A_0}{B}\right\}.$$

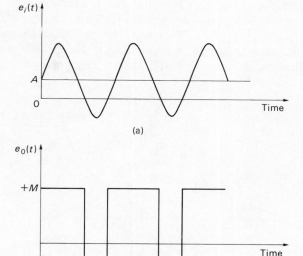

(a)

(b)

FIG. 5.10. (a) Sinusoidal input to the non-linearity superimposed on a d.c. offset. (b) Output from the non-linearity due to the input shown in (a).

Hence $e_0(t)$ will be positive for $2\cos^{-1}\left(\dfrac{-A_0}{B}\right)$ out of the cycle (2π). Therefore the average value for $e_0(t)$ in its positive phase is $M \cdot 2\cos^{-1}\left\{\dfrac{-A_0}{B}\right\}$, and for its negative phase $-M\left\{2\pi - 2\cos^{-1}\left(\dfrac{-A_0}{B}\right)\right\}$.

The average value of $e_0(t)$ is therefore:

$$e_0(t)_{av} = \frac{2M}{\pi}\left\{\frac{-\pi}{2} + \cos^{-1}\left(\frac{A_0}{B}\right)\right\}$$

$$= \frac{2M}{\pi}\sin^{-1}\frac{A_0}{B}. \tag{5.4}$$

and the equivalent gain

$$K(A_0, B) = \frac{2M}{\pi A_0}\sin^{-1}\frac{A_0}{B}. \tag{5.5}$$

The effect on the characteristic of the non-linearity can be determined from (5.4) for different values of B. With B as a parameter, the input $e_i(t)$ is effectively A_0. Fig. 5.11 illustrates the modified characteristic for $M = \pm 1$ with constraints as defined above. Hence the effect of the external stimulus is to modify the switch elements characteristic and

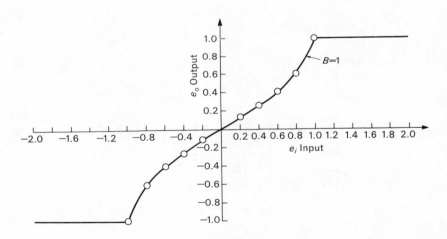

FIG. 5.11. The modified characteristic of the switch element resulting from the application of an external stimulus.

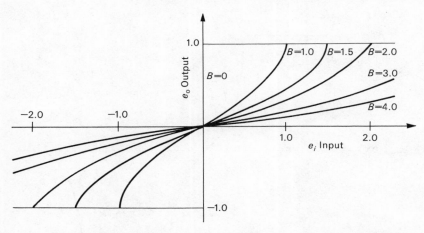

Fɪɢ. 5.12. Modified characteristics of the switch element for different magnitudes of external stimuli.

therefore its output waveform. The modified characteristics (Fig. 5.12) are used to determine the equivalent gain of the non-linearity for the DIDF in a similar manner to the single input describing function. The natural oscillation of the system $A \sin \omega t$, is applied to the appropriate modified switch element characteristic. It is important to note that the scaling of these characteristics is dependent upon the average value of the input and the modified output $e_0(t)$ obtained. Consider the cause of $B = 1$. The modified output is given by

$$e_0(0) = A \sin \theta \cdot \frac{2M}{\pi A_0} \sin^{-1} \frac{A_0}{B}. \tag{5.6}$$

If $A = 1 \cdot 57$ and A_0 (equal to e_0) lies in the range $0 \leqslant A_0 \leqslant 2 \cdot 0$, then substituting values for A_0 in eqn (5.4) gives the values shown below:

A_0	0·2	0·4	0·8	1·0	1·5	2·0
e_0	0·13	0·26	0·6	1·0	1·0	1·0

Figs. 5.12 and 5.13 illustrate the modified characteristics of the non-linear element and the output waveform, respectively.

The final step in obtaining the DIDF is to divide the fundamental component of the modified output of the non-linear element by the input due to the system, i.e. the appropriate value of A. Hence for a particular value of B the value of the equivalent gain K_{NL} can be calculated for various values of A. The family of curves produced by this calculation is

99

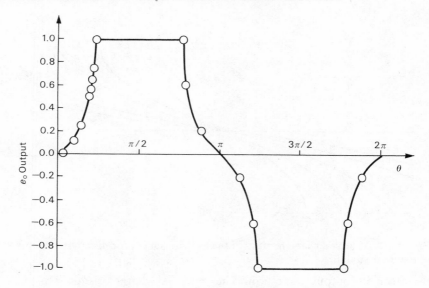

FIG. 5.13. An example of a modified output waveform from the switch element resulting from the application of an external stimulus.

illustrated in a slightly stylized form in Fig. 5.14. Referring to Fig. 5.14, the curve for $B = 0$ could have been obtained directly from the single input describing function $K_{NL} = 4M/\pi A$, e.g. when $A = 2$, $K_{NL} = 0.65$, etc.

Application of the DIDF to the model

Earlier in the chapter, the condition for a sustained oscillation was found to be $K_{NL} G(j\omega) = -1$. Hence, for the linear part of the model it is clear from eqn (5.3) that the frequency of oscillation is independent of the gain $K(22.0)$ and that with a range of K-values the conditions for stable oscillation will be maintained. However, referring to Fig. 5.14, it is clear that when an external stimulus is applied the equivalent gain of the non-linearity is reduced and a point will be reached where the natural oscillation will cease. In the model the natural frequency for a 3.3-s time delay was found to be 0.1 Hz. From eqn (5.1), the modulus of $G(j\omega)$ is

$$|G(j\omega)| = 22\left(\frac{1 + 144\omega^2}{(1 + 8464^2)(1 + 4\omega^2)}\right)^{\frac{1}{2}}. \tag{5.7}$$

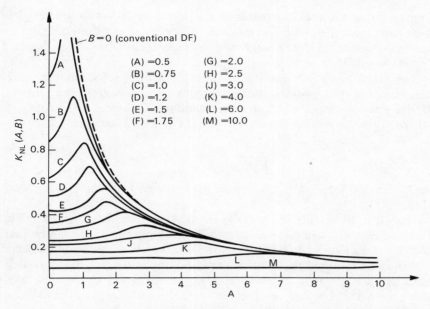

Fɪɢ. 5.14. Dual input describing function characteristics for the switch element.

The solution of eqn (5.3) gives a value for ω of $0\cdot63$; therefore substituting this value in eqn (5.6) $G(j\omega) = 1\cdot8$ and K_{NL} is $0\cdot56$. Thus referring to Fig. 5.14, a value of B of 1.4 will result in the whole of the DIDF being below the critical value of $0\cdot56$. Hence, this value will quench the natural oscillation of the system and cause the system output to comprise the external stimulus alone. This is the condition of entrainment.

The conditions for entrainment derived from the DIDF

The conditions which are required to quench a particular oscillation can be calculated on the basis of the DIDF. Consider first the case of the single input describing function where K_{NL} was found to be equal to $4M/\pi A$ for $B = 0$. (This equation generates the rectangular hyperbola shown in Fig. 5.14.) Hence no matter what the value of the equivalent gain there will always be an intersection with the locus of the linear part of the model and hence a stable limit cycle. In reality, the non-linearity has an equivalent gain which is determined from the DIDF. For the model, the crossing point of the switch element with $G(j\omega)$ was found to occur at $\omega = 0\cdot63$ rad s^{-1} and $|G(j\omega)| = 1\cdot8$. Referring to Fig. 5.14, it is

101

apparent that the oscillation will be quenched by B-values greater than 1·5. Also, once the oscillation has been quenched, the system operates on the $A = 0$ axis (Fig. 5.14) and hence a value significantly lower than 1·5 ($\approx 1\cdot1$) is sufficient to hold entrainment.

The stability of entrainment can therefore be studied on this basis. Johnson (1961) suggested a convenient graphical method for this purpose. If the system output is Y and the stimulus Z then $Z = B_c + B_c K_{NL} G$ where B_c is the critical value of B and, as $B_c K_{NL}$ is constant

$$\frac{R}{B_c K_{NL}} = \frac{1}{K_{NL}} + G,$$

and hence the value $R/B_c K_{NL}$ can be read directly from the Nyquist locus (Fig. 5.8).

From the locus (Fig. 5.7) $1/K_{NL} = 1\cdot8$; therefore, $K_{NL_{max}} = 0\cdot56$. The value of B which will provide this maximum equivalent gain can be read directly from Fig. 5.14: $B = 1\cdot5$. Once the oscillation has been quenched the B-value required to maintain this condition is $B = 1\cdot1$ the equivalent gain being $K_{NL} = 0\cdot76$. Therefore, $1/K_{NL} = 1\cdot3$ and $B_c K_{NL} = 0\cdot84$. Now using the method of Johnson the values of R for different values of ω can be calculated; these are shown in Table 5.1.

Fig. 5.15 illustrates the conditions for stable entrainment. Referring to Fig. 5.15, the characteristic defines the boundary between the stable region where entrainment exists and the unstable region where the natural frequency of oscillation of the system and the stimulus interact. The characteristic shows clearly that there is a region (here 0·4–1·2 rad s^{-1}) around the natural frequency of oscillation where the size of

TABLE 5.1

Values of R for different values of ω

	ω						
	0·01	0·02	0·05	0·15	0·2	0·29	0·38
$R/B_c K_{NL}$	15·8	11·5	7	3·8	3·2	2·6	2·2
R	13·3	9·7	5·9	3·2	2·7	2·2	1·8

	ω						
	0·55	0·63	0·73	0·82	1·0	1·2	1·56	2·0
$R/B_c K_{NL}$	0·8	0·5	0·65	1·0	1·9	2·2	2·1	3·1
R	0·67	0·42	0·55	0·84	1·6	1·8	1·76	2·6

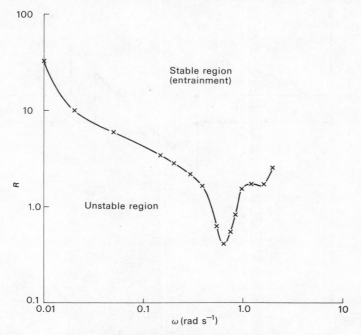

Fɪɢ. 5.15. Conditions for stable entrainment.

the stimulus required to maintain entrainment reduces dramatically, this is equivalent to the range of entrainment, described earlier in the text.

5.5. The relationship between metastable and unstable entrainment

A phenomenon which is often observed in the experimental data is that of the HRV waveform oscillating between metastable and unstable entrainment. In the introductory section the three types of entrainment (Fig. 5.1) were discussed in relation to a spontaneously oscillating non-linear system of natural frequency ω_2. In practice, the frequency of the output, in this case the thermal component of the HRV waveform, is not entirely stable and it is this instability which provides a plausible explanation for the transition phenomenon.

Fig. 5.16 illustrates the relationship between stimulus frequency and natural frequency. Let us assume that the applied stimulus is of frequency f_{STIM_1} and $f_{NAT_2} \leqslant f_{NAT} \leqslant f_{NAT_1}$. For these conditions the stimulus frequency always lies within the range of entrainment (the sloping section of

103

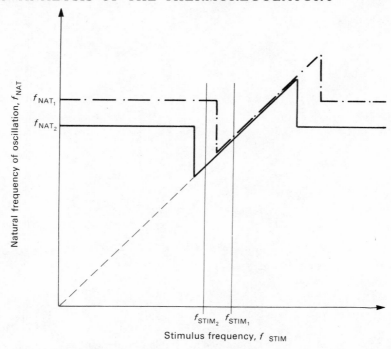

Fɪɢ. 5.16. The relationship between stimulus frequency and the natural frequency of oscillation of a non-linear biological system.

the characteristic) and the system always resides in the metastable state. If, however, the stimulus frequency is f_{STIM_2} then it can be seen from the diagram that as the natural frequency of oscillation shifts from f_{NAT_2} to f_{NAT_1} a point is reached where f_{STIM_2} lies outside the range of entrainment. Hence depending on the instantaneous value of the natural frequency the system will move in and out of entrainment. This is the condition of unstable entrainment. The interesting question is, of course, what is the physiological origin of the instability in the natural frequency of oscillation?

Heart-rate variability has been studied, using the model described in the previous section, in order to investigate the origin of the variability in the natural frequency of oscillation. The parameters of the model were systematically varied, i.e. the time constants and the pure time delay. The results showed that wide variations in the time constants produced only a minor difference in the frequency of oscillation. Whereas, even relatively minor changes in the time delay caused large changes in the frequency of oscillation. Our conclusion therefore is that the variability in the frequency of the thermal component arises from fluctuations in the pure time delay. In their paper Scher and Young (1963) describe the response of the smooth muscle comprising the peripheral resistance by a first order differential equation incorporating pure time delay. On this basis, therefore, the physiological origin of the fluctuations in the natural frequency of the thermal component of the HRV waveform would seem to be variations in the time delay associated with the response of the peripheral smooth muscle.

5.6. Conclusion

The results of our investigation which have been described can be summarized as follows:

(a) The spontaneous heart-rate variability waveform has a thermal component in the region of 0·05 Hz.
(b) The thermal component can be entrained by a periodic thermal stimulus of suitable amplitude and frequency.
(c) The entrainment phenomenon for the thermal component of the HRV waveform can be divided into three types: stable, metastable, and unstable entrainment.
(d) Continuous movement of the system between metastable and unstable entrainment seems to result from fluctuations in the natural frequency.
(e) The physiological origin of these fluctuations may be due to changes in a pure time delay associated with the characteristics of the peripheral vascular smooth muscle.

Acknowledgement

This work has been supported by the Science Research Council.

References

Boyer, R. C. (1960). Sinusoidal signal stabilisation. M.S. Thesis, Purdue University.

Burton, A. C. and Taylor, R. M. (1940). A study of the adjustment of peripheral vascular tone to the requirements of the regulation of body temperature. *Am. J. Physiol.* **129,** 565–77.

Gibson, J. E. (1963). *Nonlinear automatic control.* McGraw-Hill, New York.

Grodins, F. (1963). *Control theory and biological systems.* Columbia University Press, New York.

HATAKEGAMA, I. (1967). Analysis of baroreceptor control of the circulation. In *The physical basis of circulatory transport: regulation and exchange* (eds A. C. Guyton and E. B. Reeve). Saunders, Philadelphia, Pennsylvania.

HYNDMAN, B. W. (1970). A digital simulation of the human cardio-vascular system and its use in the study of sinus arrhythmia. Ph.D. Thesis, London University (Imperial College).

——, KITNEY, R. I., and SAYERS, B. McA. (1971). Spontaneous rhythms in physiological controls systems. *Nature,* **233** (5318) 339–41.

JOHNSON, C. D. (1961). Control and information systems laboratory memo., Purdue University. (cited by Gibson).

KITNEY, R. I. (1972). The thermoregulatory control system in man and its study by digital computer simulation. Ph.D. Thesis, London University (Imperial College).

—— (1975). An analysis of the nonlinear behaviour of the human thermal vasomotor control system. *J. theor. Biol.* **52,** 231–48.

——, ROMPELMAN, O., and SPRUYT, A. (1976). The analysis of stable and unstable oscillations in heart rate variability. *Proceedings of the 11th International Conference on Medical and Biological Engineering, Ottawa.*

—— —— (1977). Some aspects of heart rate variability. In *Biomedical computing* (ed. J. Perkins). Pitman Medical, London.

KUO, B. C. (1967). *Automatic control systems.* Prentice-Hall, Englewood Cliffs, New Jersey.

LEVISON, W. H., BARNET, G. O., and JACKSON, W. D. (1966). Nonlinear analysis of the baroreceptor reflex system. *Circ. Res.* **18,** 673.

MINORSKY, N. (1962). *Nonlinear oscillations.* Van Nostrand, Princeton, New Jersey.

ROSENBAUM, M. and RICE, D. (1968). Frequency response characteristics of the vascular resistance vessels. *Am. J. Physiol.* **215,** 1397.

SAYERS, B. McA. (1973). Analysis of heart rate variability. *Ergonom.* **16**(1), 17–32.

SCHER, A. M. and YOUNG, A. C. (1963). Servoanalysis of the carotid sinus reflex effects on peripheral resistance. *Circulation Res.* **12**(2), 152–62.

SPICKLER, J. W., KEZDI, P., and GELLER, E. (1967). Transfer characteristics of the carotid sinus pressure control system. In *Baroreceptors and hypertension* (ed. P. Kedzi). Pergamon Press, Oxford.

6.

The physiology of heart-rate control by arterial baroreceptors in man and animals

P. SLEIGHT

6.1. Introduction

IN this chapter I shall attempt a simplified description of the nervous control of arterial pressure. For a full review of the literature to about 1972–3 there is a comprehensive account by Kircheim (1976); Korner (1971) deals with central integration of the baroreflexes with other nervous inputs; shorter accounts with more recent references are given by Sleight (1974, 1976).

This volume is devoted to the topic of heart-rate control. Without wishing to deny the time-honoured convenience of expressing the heart frequency in beats/min, I hope I can convince the reader of the greater ease of control analysis which comes from expressing it as pulse interval (ms). It has long been known that when the blood-pressure is disturbed from its normal level the heart slows down or speeds up in an attempt to return the pressure to the control value or 'set' point. The relation between pressure and rate is curvilinear but that between pressure and interval is linear, at any rate for pressures around the normal value.

For each heartbeat the arterial pressure rapidly (in about 100 ms) reaches a peak (the systolic pressure) and then declines to a trough (the diastolic pressure). Mean pressure may be obtained by integration or, frequently, by adding one-third of the pulse pressure to the diastolic pressure. All three can be used as the input to the control system but in practice we have used only the systolic pressure as an index of the stimulus. We have found that in man there is a reliable linear correlation between the systolic pressure of one beat and the pulse interval (ms) which follows before the next beat, provided that the subject is in a steady state (Fig. 6.1).

The relation is rapidly altered or 'reset' by any disturbance whether mental (anxiety, mental arithmetic) or physical (posture, exercise). After such a change in state the gain of the reflex arc is altered to a new value.

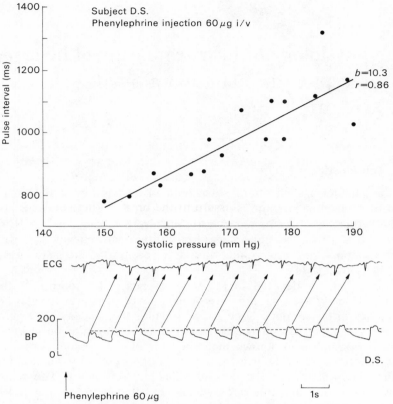

Fɪɢ. 6.1. Lower panel shows the brachial artery blood-pressure (BP) (mm Hg) and electrocardiogram recorded in a subject shortly after the intravenous injection of 60 μg of phenylephrene. The arrows show the pulse intervals with which the prior systolic pressures have been correlated. The plot in the upper panel is derived from this data. The slope 10·3 ms mm Hg^{-1} gives a numerical index of the baroreflex gain for heart-rate control. (From Sleight, Gribbin, and Pickering 1971.)

There is also a concomitant change in the 'set' point for pressure or pulse interval.

6.2. Historical review

Although the existence of accelerator and depressor nerves to the heart had been demonstrated by electrical stimulation more than 100 years ago, and although it had been suspected that these nerves were regulated by the pressure in the heart, it was not until the mid-1920s that Hering described the importance of the carotid sinus as the nervous input of the control system. The carotid sinus is a localized dilatation at the beginning of the internal carotid artery, where it leaves the main carotid artery at the angle of the jaw. The internal carotid then penetrates the skull to form a major blood supply to the brain. The fibrous outer coat (adventitia) of the sinus is richly supplied with nerve endings which signal stretch of the wall (and thus, indirectly, pressure).

The wall of the sinus is more elastic and more distensible than the arterial wall on either side and we have found that it responds rapidly and faithfully to changes in transmural pressure with minimal creep and minimal hysteresis. It is positioned very strategically to monitor and maintain an adequate supply pressure to the brain. Other similar stretch receptors have been found in the aorta and heart.

6.3. Receptor physiology

Since 1932 it has been possible to record the small currents which are excited in the carotid sinus nerve after stimulation of the receptors. At pressures around normal the nerve output gives an extremely accurate record of the arterial wave form (Fig. 6.2). However the receptors exhibit

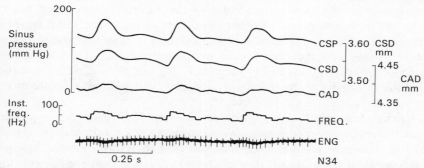

FIG. 6.2. Records (from an anaesthetized greyhound), read from the top down. Pressure in the carotid sinus (CSP); carotid sinus diameter (CSD) measured by ultrasound transit time, (from minute crystals pocketed in the fibrous sheath of the sinus); carotid artery diameter (CAD), which follows the pressure changes less faithfully; and the instantaneous firing frequency of the single baroreceptor fibre whose action potentials are shown as the lowest trace. (From Bergel, D., Brooks, D. E., MacDermott, A. J., Robinson, J. L., and Sleight, P. unpublished observations.)

109

a threshold which is very variable: e.g. ranging from about 60 to 130 mm Hg in the normal dog, and even higher in hypertensive animals. The nerve output is linear above this threshold, when plotted against pressure. At higher pressures however (about 170 mm Hg) the response rapidly flattens out and reaches a plateau. We have recently shown that this can be explained by the increasing stiffness, and hence decreasing stretch, of the sinus wall (Bergel, Brooks, MacDermott, Robinson, and Sleight 1976).

The receptors respond in a complex but predictable way to changes in pressure. They are influenced by the absolute level of pressure and also by the rate of change of pressure and by the pulse pressure. They are also influenced of course by the frequency of the heart beat.

These same characteristics of the receptor input to the system are closely followed by the output so that the full stimulus response curve is S-shaped with a threshold, a linear portion, and a plateau. We have developed a method of baroreflex testing in man which we have been using for the last 10 years (Smyth, Sleight, and Pickering 1969). We use a vasoconstrictor drug phenylephrine, injected intravenously in a dose of 50–150 μg. This causes a temporary (about 1 min) rise in arterial pressure of 20–30 mm Hg.

During the rising phase of pressure we plot the relation between systolic pressure and the succeeding pulse interval. The slope of the linear regression gives a quantitative index of the baroreflex control of heart-rate. We do not measure the other motor arm of the reflex, but it appears from studies of carotid sinus nerve stimulation in man that the response of heart-rate and the response of peripheral vascular dilatation (sympathetic withdrawal) are rather parallel. Using this method we have found that the sensitivity of the reflex arc diminishes with patients who are older or who have high blood pressure.

Critics of the method (e.g. Kidd and Linden 1975) have been worried that the sensitivity of the reflex as we measure it appears closely related to the resting or control pulse interval. It is therefore of some interest (and personal satisfaction!) that Eckberg (1977) has come to the conclusion that the resting pulse interval in man is determined by the baroreflex gain and not vice versa. We have found that the gain of the reflex for heart-rate (pulse interval) control is greatest during sleep. It is depressed during exercise.

It is interesting that the gain is increased by clonidine, a drug used in the treatment of hypertension. This drug stimulates α-adrenergic receptors, which are the receptors which primarily respond to noradrenaline, and might therefore be expected to cause peripheral vaso-constriction and hence hypertension. From animal experiments it seems likely that clonidine acts primarily in the central nervous system (CNS). Here, paradoxically, α-adrenergic stimulation depresses peripheral nervous sympathetic tone. We have found (Sleight, West, Korner, Oliver, Chalmers, and Robinson 1975) that minute doses of clonidine ($0\cdot05-1\cdot5$ μg) injected into the lateral cerebral ventricle of rabbits markedly increased the gain of the baroreflex arc. It appears that this effect is probably responsible for its hypotensive action in man.

The major disputed question at present is whether the baroreceptors have any important influences or long-term control of the level of arterial blood-pressure in man or animals. Guyton and his colleagues (Cowley, Liard, and Guyton 1973) have questioned this. They cut the nerves from the principal arterial receptors in dogs and then measured the blood-pressure over 24 h, in much the same way as we have measured in man (Littler, Honour, Sleight, and Stott 1972).

They found that *when the dogs were isolated* (our italics) the blood-pressure over 24 h, although extremely variable, was on average only a few mm Hg higher than before cutting the nerves. They inferred from this that long-term control of arterial pressure was not dependent on baroreflexes.

This question is unresolved but our own data would be in conflict with Guyton's view. We have seen subjects who have for other reasons sustained damage to the carotid sinus receptors. These subjects commonly develop high blood-pressure. We have already shown that environmental factors impair the sensitivity of the baroreflex and we therefore believe that Guyton's experiments, although of great interest, are not really relevant to man, since the animals were isolated from environmental stimuli. We believe that it is naive to think of the baroreflex as being divorced from these influences since we already know that it can be 'reset' by such stimuli. If the animal has impaired reflexes because of surgical denervation, it seems likely that environmental stimuli could then act to cause hypertension.

Man is unique amongst animals in his susceptibility to arterial degeneration. This is particularly so at arterial branches and the carotid sinus is one of the most seriously affected areas in the arterial tree. Heath and his colleagues (Winson, Heath, and Smith 1974) have shown the progressive deterioration in the carotid sinus with age in man. I believe that this impairment, plus the influence of environmental changes acting through the mind, could be important factors in the development and progression of essential hypertension.

111

6.4. Conclusion

The physiology of the baroreflex arc controlling heart-rate is reviewed. When the blood-pressure is perturbed during a previous steady state there is a linear relation between systolic blood-pressure and pulse interval. The slope of this relation can be used as a quantitative measure of the gain of the reflex arc. Gain is greatest during sleep, particularly dreams, and it is diminished by upright posture and even more so by exercise or mental activity.

Certain drugs, such as clonidine, probably have their therapeutic action by increasing the gain of the baroreflex arc by an action in the central nervous system.

High blood-pressure in man may be partly related to increasing stiffness of the arterial wall where the sensory receptors lie.

References

BERGEL, D. H., BROOKS, D. E., MacDERMOTT, A. J., ROBINSON, J. L., and SLEIGHT, P. (1976). The relation between carotid sinus dimension, nerve activity and pressure in the anaesthetised greyhound. *J. Physiol.* **263**, 156–7P.

COWLEY, A. W., LIARD, J. F., and GUYTON, A. C. (1973). Role of the baroreceptor reflex in daily control of arterial blood pressure and other variables in dogs. *Circulation Res.* **32**, 564–76.

ECKBERG, D. L. (1977). Baroreflex inhibition of the human sinus node: importance of stimulus intensity, duration, and rate of pressure change. *J. Physiol.* **269**, 561–77.

KIDD, C. and LINDEN, R. J. (1975). Recent advances in the physiology of cardiovascular reflexes, with special reference to hypotension. *Br. J. Anaesthesia* **47**, 767–76.

KIRCHEIM, H. R. (1976). Systemic arterial baroreceptor reflexes. *Physiol. Rev.* **56**, 100–76.

KORNER, P. I. (1971). Integrative neural cardiovascular control. *Physiol. Rev.* **51**, 312–29.

LITTLER, W. A., HONOUR, A. J., SLEIGHT, P., and STOTT, F. D. (1972). Continuous recording of direct arterial blood pressure and electrocardiogram in unrestricted man. *Br. med. J.* **iii**, 76–8.

SLEIGHT, P. (1974). Neural control of the cardiovascular system. In *Modern trends in cardiology* (ed. M. F. Oliver), pp. 1–43. Butterworths, London.

—— (1976). Neurophysiology of the carotid sinus receptors in normal and hypertensive animals and man. *Cardiology* **61** (Suppl. 1), 31–45.

——, GRIBBIN, B., and PICKERING, T. G. (1971). Baroreflex sensitivity in normal and hypertensive man; the effect of beta-adrenergic blockade on reflex sensitivity. *Postgrad. med. J.* **47**, (Suppl.), p. 79.

——, ROBINSON, J. L., BROOKS, D., and REES, P. M. (1977). Characteristics of single carotid sinus baroreceptor fibres and whole nerve activity in the normotensive and the renal hypertensive dog. *Circulation Res.* **41,** 750–8.

——, WEST, M. J., KORNER, P. I., OLIVER, J. R., CHALMERS, J. P. and ROBINSON, J. L. (1975). The action of clonidine on the baroreflex control of heart rate in conscious animals and man, and on single aortic baroreceptor discharge in the rabbit. *Arch. int. Pharmacodynam.* **214,** 4–11.

SMYTH, H. S., SLEIGHT, P., and PICKERING, G. W. (1969). Reflex regulation of the arterial pressure during sleep in man: a quantitative method of assessing baroreflex sensitivity. *Circulation Res.* **24,** 109–21.

WINSON, M., HEATH, D., and SMITH, P. (1974). Extensibility of the human carotid sinus. *Cardiovasc. Res.* **8,** 58–64.

Part IV

Other aspects of heart-rate variability analysis

7.
Heart-rate and its variability—pitfalls, etc.
G. H. Byford

7.1. Introduction

We learn from the daily press that young school teachers are under stress when dealing with fractious classes; classes in which books are amongst an armoury of student missiles and desk lids are so misemployed as to add to auditory pollution of the classroom. Elsewhere in the same publications we are enjoined to travel by Inter-city train and thereby avoid the competition and stress of travelling by car. The evidence upon which these views are based is that heart-rate increases under those supposedly adverse conditions, and ergo, that is a bad thing; no statistical questions appear to have been asked of that evidence and no statistical answers are given; moreover it appears that the conclusions are drawn as a result of comparisons between unlike and unlike, a procedure of doubtful scientific validity. That the heart should change its rate of beating may come as no surprise: indeed it might almost be said that we should be more upset if its beat did not vary, since there are perfectly reasonable mechanisms which are intended to ensure that it does so. The cost of acquiring such data over long periods and the effort which is spent in obtaining it, might lead us to ask what is the purpose behind such investigations when we know that a heart which beats for relatively short periods at up to 200 beats min^{-1} may well be behaving quite normally.

Before heart-rate measurements can be shown to be useful in the assessment of stress, it is necessary first to assure ourselves that changes in rate are indeed indications of some undesirable psychological or physiological state, and then to establish a correlation between heart-rate and those consequences of stress which we believe are best avoided: it is not enough simply to establish that heart-rate changes are accompanied by changes in stress—there are a great many pleasurable but stressful reasons why heart-rate should increase.

7.2. Problems in using ECG measurements

One of the of the least difficult of electrophysiological recordings is the ECG—it requires no sophisticated equipment and little specialist knowledge so long as nothing more than approximate rate is required; but if at some stage there might be the need for a clinical interpretation of the electrocardiogram, then clearly it has to be recorded in accordance with the standards common in clinical medicine, and that in some situations may not be quite so simple. In order to measure rate accurately we must first establish some part of the R wave as a fiducial point from which the interval between one R wave and the next is to be measured; having done this we may develop an algorithm to proceed in a logical fashion with our measurement and the subsequent calculations. If we are unable accurately to locate the R peak then we are faced with a source of variability, about which we know little, but which nevertheless contributes to our inability to obtain the best from our recordings. Consider the high-speed examples of the R wave of Fig. 7.1, taken from a 1 min electrocardiogram recorded from a normal subject under normal conditions. The bandwidth of that recording is in excess of 100 Hz, and the indecision surrounding what might be loosely called the 'peak' is clearly evident, but it might be argued that we have no need of this bandwidth; why not introduce a low-pass filter. That would certainly remove the symptoms—it would also leave the disease unchecked and us in a fool's R-wave paradise: the unavoidable non-linear phase changes would add to our uncertainty.

It needs but a few very simple experiments to demonstrate that heart-rate changes, during the respiratory cycle, with posture, and with psychological state; and depending upon electrode site and other factors, the ECG itself may change in shape. The physiological events reflected by the changing potential are such that although the peak of the R wave may at one time represent a stable point in the cardiac cycle, under different conditions the recorded peak will no longer represent the same physiological point (Fig. 7.2). That the heart is quite clearly capable of changing its rate extremely rapidly can convincingly be demonstrated by placing a subject in a human centrifuge and plotting RR intervals as a function of time whilst the subject is undergoing an increased gravitational stress—Fig. 7.3 illustrates this and needs no further explanation. It has also been shown (Dornhorst, Howard, and Leathart 1952) that under certain conditions Tauber waves, at approximately 4 min^{-1}, can be detected: these waves result in cyclic variations of blood-pressure and heart-rate. Of course not all these potential problems will be present at

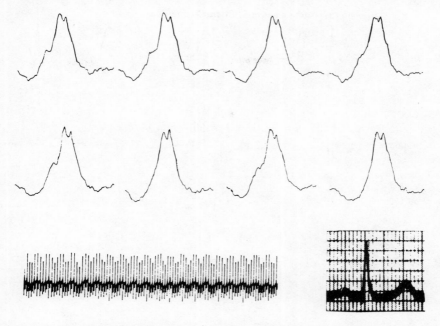

FIG. 7.1. The R wave. What constitutes the R wave peak and what algorithm can be used to detect it *unambiguously*?. The upper eight examples are from a high-speed recording, and although this detail is not normally visible, it is present when an electrical signal is automatically digitized. *Lower left*: the respiratory artefact in R wave amplitude; a similar unwanted variation affects the RR interval. *Lower right*: the ECG as seen by textbooks of physiology.

one and the same time, but it is difficult to be certain in advance even with the most carefully prepared experimental situation, that none of them are present, or if they are, what their effect will be. Our aim therefore is to minimize as far as possible any source of variability which is not directly due to the problem with which we are concerned.

7.3. Problems in statistical analysis of heart-rate

The expression 'heart-rate' can be misleading, and 'instantaneous rate' even more misleading: rate necessarily implies that a measurement has been made for a number of beats, and this may not be the case; even if it were, rapid changes in rate would be masked by the averaging process—'RR interval' is a more suitable label. It has already been pointed out that

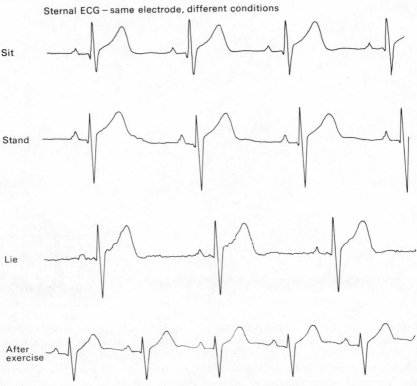

Fig. 7.2. The ECG recorded under different conditions: the 'peak' is not easily defined; filtering the signal may introduce frequency-dependent delays and do no more than exchange one problem for another.

the RR interval may vary for a variety of reasons, and that it may not itself be of great value, and there is a body of opinion which suggests that the variability of this measure contains information useful to investigators. We are required then to find some numerical description for variability, together with a technique which will enable us to establish the existence of the probable differences between two variabilities. If the data were 'normally distributed' there are several statistical techniques of a relatively elementary nature which would be adequate for the purpose. Unfortunately this statistical Utopia does not always exist and we are faced with the possibility that the data is distributed in some other way, that it is probably non-stationary, and that much of its variation is due to

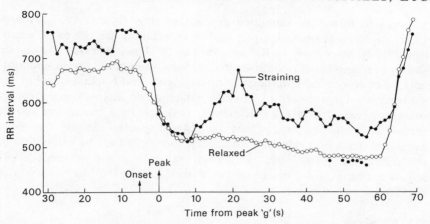

FIG. 7.3. Changes in RR interval whilst a subject is seated in a centrifuge. Note the very rapid recovery at the 60-s point, where the centrifuge comes rapidly to rest.

cyclic factors of both specific and non-specific origin. It is just these cyclic factors which from time to time have been the inspiration for attempts to produce spectral estimates from RR-interval data.

The presence of variability which changes in some cyclic manner outside the already known periodic changes of heart-rate, is evidence for the existence of information that could be of value. However, spectral estimates, whilst they are simple to calculate, are not so simple to interpret. The single raw estimates calculated with the aid of the fast Fourier transform, or autocorrelation, provide insufficient degrees of freedom on which to base a statistical test of significance; it may therefore be necessary to collect more data than textbook theory would suggest, in order that practical value can be extracted from the recordings. We have next to decide whether that statistical significance test is to be made between two spectral estimates at the same frequency but taken on different occasions, or between two complete spectra, again taken on different occasions. Power spectral densities and similar measures are based on assumptions, and it is only with extreme care that one can avoid violating those assumptions, the principal one of which is that the data shall be stationary over the period of the measurement—this in general is patently untrue. To venture into the realms of non-stationary time series analysis would undoubtedly involve conflict since this special branch of complex statistics is not yet well documented and in spite of several

121

attempts to introduce simplified procedures (e.g. Byford 1977; Adams 1977), agreement on techniques and interpretation has yet to be established. If cyclic changes in RR interval can be shown to exist, and can be shown to change under controlled conditions, the matter would undoubtedly be of considerable interest to physiologists and to clinicians, but the evidence so far appears to be that whilst cyclic changes are strongly suggested, no objective experimental evidence of a numerical nature seems to be forthcoming. Once the power spectral density has been estimated it is but a relatively short step to proceed to the estimation of the coherence, phase, and gain. Their value may not be immediately apparent but these factors could be of assistance in the interpretation of the data.

7.4. Conclusion

There can be no doubt that variations in the heart's rate, whether they be short- or long-term, have potential diagnostic value, but we have yet to show what that value is. Some of the precise analytical tools now being brought to bear on this subject are powerful, very powerful; their use can be justified only by competent data and by an understanding adequate to make their precision valuable. Merely to confirm by an elaborate instrumentational procedure, that which is already known without recourse to additional experimentation, is surely no way to spend our valuable resources, and we might consider with concern the possibility that ill-considered studies of heart-rate and its variability could bring disrepute to the subject before its contributions have been properly assessed.

References

ADAMS, E. R. (1977). Some new digital techniques for the analysis of non-stationary time series. *Proceedings Colloquium on Applications of Time Series Analysis*. University of Southampton.

BYFORD, G. H. (1977). Dynamic spectral comparisons for non-stationary data. *Proceedings IEE Colloquium on Random Signal Analysis*.

DORNHORST, A. C., HOWARD, P., and LEATHART, G. L. (1952). Respiratory variations in blood pressure. *Circulation* **6**(4),

8.

Decomposition of heart-rate variability under the ergonomic aspects of stressor analysis

H. LUCZAK, U. PHILIPP, AND W. ROHMERT

8.1. Introduction: scales of heart-rate variation

IN this chapter we are concerned with the measurement of heart-rate variation for the ergonomic purpose of evaluating strain in human operators in practical working situations. A problem immediately arises: what kind of variation in *noise* (using the word in the communications engineering sense) and what kind of variation in *signal* is a meaningful phenomenon, which allows interpretation and has practical consequences? The ergonomic analysis of this problem leads to the conclusion that the signal-to-noise ratio in heart-rate variation is largely dependent on the research objectives of the experimenter, i.e. on what kind and what amount of workload is being studied. The problem has two aspects: (1) the kind of stressors acting as stimuli, i.e. stressor variation (Monod 1967; Rohmert, Laurig, Philipp, and Luczak 1973), and (2) the *scale of* frequency response of a time series of heart-rate measurements.

Using the scale of frequency response as a guideline for a classification of heart-rate variation, the effects within the certain frequency bands can be assigned to the signal and to the noise side, taking into account that what is signal in one band is noise in another. For the evaluation of physical workload, for instance, the high-frequency components due to rhythmic variations have a disturbance effect (Monod 1967), and for the evaluation of non-physical strain any muscular-induced low-frequency variation masks, in a nearly uncontrollable manner, the components of higher frequency which might have an interpretative value for this type of strain (Rohmert *et al.* 1973). Spectral analyses by various workers (Sayers 1973; Luczak and Laurig 1973; Hyndman and Gregory 1975) have shown that the cardiac interbeat interval signal contains information in the range from 0 to 0·5 Hz. In this range exogenous and endogenous, intra- and inter-individual, autorhythmic and imposition/entrainment-induced variations occur (Monod 1967; Sayers 1973).

Within range I, i.e. 0 to $0·5 \times 10^{-4}$ Hz—the annual as well as the diurnal scale—seasonal variations with respect to supposedly thermoregulatory mechanisms occur (Renbourn 1962): an ergonomic evaluation of shift-regimes tells us that the diurnal cycles and the sleep effects (Engel, Hildebrandt, and Vogt 1969) can be considered as signal, whereas the variations due to pregnancy, training, and the seasonal effects mentioned above might be noise within this context.

From 0.5×10^{-4} to 0.5×10^{-2} Hz—the range II of heart-rate changes—there is expansion within the scale of shift-time. Here destabilization effects of the cardio-respiratory system can be measured which can be attributed to fatigue, mainly caused by physical load (Rohmert 1960, 1962) characterized by various types of muscular and environmental stressors (Monod 1967). Variations in this range which can be accounted to non-physical causes, such as adaptation processes (Rutenfranz, Rohmert, and Iskander 1971) and mental work above endurance limits (Rohmert and Luczak 1973), can also be filtered out.

In range III, from 0.5×10^{-2} to 0.5×10^{-1} Hz, can be placed the direct reaction of heart-rate to external load situations. This can be due to changes of posture, dynamic and static work, reactions to changes in the physical and chemical environment, and the effects of psychosensory, emotional, and even mental stimuli on the operator. The pattern of this reaction is frequently specific for the type and amount of workload, but if different stressors (in the sense mentioned) are superimposed it is usually impossible to separate them because of the integrative nature of cardio-vascular and cardiorespiratory response to all these stimuli.

Range IV, extending from 0.5×10^{-1} to 0.5 Hz, is called *heart-rate variability* or arrhythmia. Besides rhythmic variations, such as are caused by variations in blood-pressure and respiration (including speaking effects), by fluctuations in vasomotor tone, and possibly by thermoregulatory waves (Sayers 1973), a reaction to the mental or information-processing activities of the human operator is supposed to exist characterized by a depression of the amplitude of the signal and a shift to higher frequencies occurring in the cardiac interbeat interval sequence, as compared with conditions of rest.

Many tasks of information-processing by a human operator are not directly connected with measurable activities of information perception or information output by the subject. In these cases, where measurement of performance is impossible or provides no information for an ergonomic assessment of the work situation, the measurement of physiological indicators of strain is the only possible means of obtaining objective information on the subject's condition when performing a task.

Attention was therefore drawn to the objective measurement of reaction to mental load by scoring heart-rate variability, initially by Wiersma (1931), Schlohmka (1936), and Malmö and Shagass (1949), and later by Bartenwerfer (1960) and Kalsbeek (1963, 1967). A broader application of heart-rate variability, or sinus arrhythmia, as a measure of mental strain is mainly connected with the development of automatic measurement techniques and appropriate computer programs. Progress in data-processing techniques led to experiments and methodological studies on heart-rate variability in laboratories in various countries (Ettema 1967; Ettema and Zielhuis 1971; Danev and Wartna 1970; Danev, Wartna, Bink, Radder, and Luteyn 1972; Wartna, Danev, and Bink 1971; Laurig and Philipp 1970; Laurig, Luczak, and Philipp 1971; Klinger and Strasser 1972) and culminated in a symposium on Heart Rate Variability of the Ergonomics Research Society in October 1971. The papers presented there were published in *Ergonomics* in 1973 (Firth 1973; Sayers 1973; Rohmert *et al.* 1973*a*; Zwaga 1973; Mulder and Mulder-Majonides 1973; Luczak and Laurig 1973; Opmeer 1973). They contain results reflecting the different research approaches of the authors in terms of theoretical concepts, scoring methods, and experimental conditions. Further experimental results were reported by Strasser (1974), Boyce (1974), and Gaillard and Trumbo (1976) whereas Hyndman and Gregory (1975) and Luczak and Raschke (1975) tried to apply theoretical systems analysis to the problem. The trend from a purely experimental and correlational approach to a more causal view of the phenomenon of 'heart-rate variability' can be observed in the literature. There is a fundamental need for a greater understanding of the complexity of physiological responses. The 'black box', generating heart-rate variability and its reaction on mental load, must be described quantitatively. According to Sayers (1973), Hyndman, Kitney, and Sayers (1971), and Pasmooy (1972), the black box can be described in three ways: first by a physiological and theoretical systems analysis of the structure and function of the cardiovascular and cardiorespiratory system with its neural implications; second by experiments which do not rely on arbitrary types of mental load, but which investigate systematically the effects on heart-rate variability of the superimposition of motor and informational, mental, and emotional components of stress; and third by an analysis of the reaction of heart-rate variability to a specific type of workload in relation to the reaction to other physiological variables, i.e. a polygraphic measurement and evaluation concept.

8.2. Research approach to heart-rate variation (HRV) in ergonomic terms

The preceding section illustrates that an appropriate high- or low-pass filtering procedure makes it possible to connect various kinds of heart-rate variation (HRV) to various ergonomic problems of evaluation. Though our further analysis within this chapter will be centred around scale IV, which is called heart-rate variability, the interference from superimposition of variations from different scales in actual recordings of instantaneous heart-rate require a thorough analysis in numerical terms using various research approaches. This is a prerequisite of ergonomic interpretation.

The approach presented in the following pages is threefold: first an analysis in terms of biomedical engineering and biological cybernetics is outlined, which tries to model the information flow in the cardio-vascular and cardio-respiratory system in terms of control theory. Second, experimental findings on the superimposition of various stressors are presented. These experiments include systematic variations in the type and amount of workload using appropriate models to assess their effect on heart-rate variability. This approach, which can be seen in the context of classical work physiology, relates external work stimuli to internal physiological reactions. Third, physiological reactions are further analyzed with the help of a concept of polygraphic measurement, in an attempt to follow the psychophysiological interdependencies, in the measurement of different frequency bands in the electroencephalogram, of catecholamine secretion and of respiratory cycles. This strain component analysis under a high stimulus of mental and emotional workload (in this case in university examinations), tries to relate the dynamics of various physiological systems to each other within the concept of arousal.

All three approaches, however, must be seen under the controlling objective of explaining HRV in relation to ergonomic purposes. Our basic aim is to interpret the relation between the external stressors and the components of strain in a human operator and to improve the applicability of HRV in evaluating practical working situations.

8.3. Analysis of a model of the cardiovascular and cardiorespiratory system

Most of the authors mentioned above have found that only a small part of scored HRV changed under conditions of mental load. The major part remains unaffected by the workload. In terms of communication theory it may be said that the signal-to-noise ratio of the measurement is very bad. To explain this 'physiological noise' means to reduce the uncertainty of measurement of HRV. The model to be described explains and interprets in a quantitative and deterministic way the effect of the main physiological functions.

Model

The model presented here is based on one published earlier by Luczak and Raschke (1975). The original version was extended to include muscular workload conditions above endurance limits—anaerobic work; in addition the mechanisms of rhythm generation and control of the frequency and amplitude of respiration and blood-pressure have been substantially revised.

The model describes the control and rhythmic genesis of instantaneous heart-rate, respiration, and blood-pressure, i.e. those physiological functions which, after spectral analyses (Sayers 1973), mainly affect heart-rate variability under rest and physical and non-physical stress conditions. The structure-block diagram of the model is shown in Fig. 8.1; the functional relationships (the system of equations referred to hereafter) are given in Table 8.1.

The generation of the rhythm of respiration can be located in the central nervous system (Feldman and Cowan 1975a, b) (eqns (8.1), (8.2), (8.3)). Rhythmic action potentials in α-neuromotor regions are produced by a sinus oscillator, variable in amplitude and frequency. The influence of the stretch receptors in the lung must be subtracted from the output of the sinus oscillator. Frequency and amplitude of respiration are functions of workload (Stegemann 1971; Horgan and Lange 1962, 1964; Hartung 1966; Piiper 1972).

The α-motorneurons affect the thoracic intercostal muscles and the diaphragm. Their behaviour is approximately described by a PT_1 transfer function (eqn 8.4). The signal of the stretch receptors in the lung is fed back to the α-neuromotor regions. Their influence is approximated by a PDT_1 function (after Keidel 1973). The constants of the stretch receptors and the thoracic and diaphragm muscles had to be approximated, because quantitative descriptions could not be found in the literature. The constants were adjusted by adapting the values of respiratory arrhythmia for high frequencies of respiration given by Angelone and Coulter (1964).

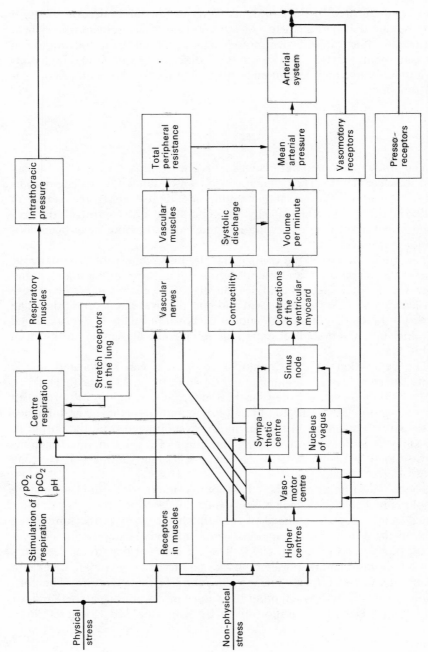

Fig. 8.1. Block diagram of physiological interactions in the cardio-vascular system, influencing HRV.

TABLE 8.1

Systems of equations for the description of the behaviour of physiological functions and their coupling in the cardio-vascular and cardio-respiratory systems—a model of heart-rate variability.

Physiological function	System of equations	Symbols, denominations, units
Generation of rhythm and amplitude of respiration (neuronal aspects of ventilation)	(8.1) $P_{VE} = P_{CRDP} - P_{Ldr}$ (8.2) $P_{CRDP} = \hat{P}_{CRDP} \cdot A \cdot \sin \omega t$ (8.3) $f_A = \omega/2\pi$	P_{VE} = rate of impulses of the α-motorneurons P_{CRDP} = Impulses of central origin A = Amplitude factor f_A = Frequency of respiration P_{Ldr} = Afferent impulses of stretch receptors in the lung
Mechanical function of lung-muscles (mechanical aspects of ventilation)	(8.4) $\dfrac{V_E}{P_{VE}} = \dfrac{K_{VE}}{1 + T_{VE} \cdot p}$	V_E = momentary value of ventilation K_{VE} = 5 (impulses s^{-1})$^{-1}$ T_{VE} = 0·2 (s)
Stretch receptors in the lung; feed-back to α-neuro-motor regions	(8.5) $\dfrac{P_{Ldr}}{V_E} = \dfrac{K_4(1 + T_5 p)}{1 + T_6 p}$	K_4 = 0·25 (impulses s^{-1}) T_5 = 2 (s) T_6 = 1 (s)
Coupling between respiration and blood-pressure	(8.6) $P_z = P_{ith}$ for $\dfrac{dP_{ith}}{dt} < 0$ (8.7) $P_z = 0$ for $\dfrac{dP_{ith}}{dt} > 0$ (8.8) $P_{ith} = K \dfrac{\tau_p \cdot p}{1 + \tau_p \cdot p}$ (8.9) $\dfrac{f_{AWph}}{W_{ph}} = K_{Wph1} \dfrac{k_f}{1 + T_f \cdot p}$	P_z = disturbance function for blood-pressure P_{ith} = pneumatic intrathoracic pressure K = 1 τ_p = 0·5 (s)

Description	Eq.	Equation	Variables
			$a = 1.74;\ b = 0.96;\ D_1 = 0.65$ $\omega_{n1} = 1\ [\text{rad s}^{-1}];\ K_{PF} = \text{constant}$
Feedback for blood-pressure regulation over receptors in the vasomotor regions	(8.14)	$\dfrac{F_{aff2}}{P_m} = k\,\dfrac{1+\tau_1 p}{1+\tau_2 p}$	F_{aff2} = Afferent impulses of the receptors for vasomotor $k = 1$ impulse s^{-1} (mm Hg)$^{-1}$ $\tau_1 = 0.1$ (s) $\tau_2 = 0.05$(s)
Behaviour of the vasomotor muscles	(8.15)	$\dfrac{K_g}{F_{effl}} = \dfrac{k_5(1+T_7 p)}{1+T_8 p}$	K_g = Status of contraction of vasomotor muscles F_{effl} = Impulses to vasomotor $k_5 = 0.998$ (s impulse^{-1}) $T_7 = 0.05$ (s); $T_8 = 0.2$ (s)
Peripheral resistance	(8.16)	$R_t = \dfrac{R_{to}}{1 + K_6 W_s - K_{11} K_g}$	R_{to} = Peripheral resistance in rest $K_6 = 0.0832$ $K_{11} = 1$
Generation of the central rhythm of blood-pressure	(8.17) (8.18)	$F_{effl} = B.\sin \omega t (K_7 . F_{aff2} + k_{10}) . K_g$ $+ K_{11} . F_{aff2}$ $f_v = K_8(K_7 . F_{aff2} + K_{10})$	$B \sin \omega t$ = Central rhythm of the vasomotor centre f_v = Frequency of the vasomotor tonus $K_7 = 0.25;\ K_3 = 0.18;\ K_8 = 0.776$ K_{10} = Constant determining the influence of the central nervous system
Regulation of increase of heart-rate by sympathetic tonization; the impulses are generated by muscle-receptors	(8.19) (8.20) (8.21) (8.22)	$W_s = \dfrac{p(1+T_2 p)Y_1 + K_{ref} W_{ph}(K_2 . p + T_1)}{T_2 p^2 + (K_2+1)p + T_1}$ with $Y_1 = \dfrac{K_w . K_1}{1+T_1 p}$ and $K_w = K_0 W_{ph}$ for $W_{ph} < W_{DLG}$ $K_w = \text{constant}$ for $W_{ph} > W_{DLG}$	$T_1 = 16$ (s) $T_2 = 23.4$ (s) $T_1 = 0.0353$ (s^{-1}) $K_1 = 0.604$ $K_2 = 0.157$ $K_{ref} = 0.0557$ W_{DLG} = Physical workload at the endurance limit

Dimensions and units are given when this is possible in physiological and physical terms; otherwise the variables can be seen as reference variables.

Physiological function		System of equations	Symbols, denominations, units
Influence of physical workload on respiration	(8.10)	$\dfrac{P_{wph}}{W_{ph}} = K_{wph2} \dfrac{k_p}{1 + T_p \cdot p}$	W_{ph} = Physical workload $K_{wph1,2}$ = Constants, dependent on physical workload f_{Awph} = Increase of frequency of respiration under physical workload P_{wph} = Influence of physical workload on the amplitude of respiration $T_f = 54$ (s) $T_p = 34.8$ (s) $k_f = k_p = 1$
'Quick' regulation of blood-pressure by cardiac output	(8.11)	$P_m = R_t \cdot Q \dfrac{\omega_{n2}}{p^2 + 2D_2\omega_{n2} \cdot p + \omega_{n2}^2}$	P_m = Mean pressure in arteries (mm Hg) R_t = peripherial resistance (mm Hg min l^{-1}) Q = cardiac output (beat min^{-1}) $\omega_{n2} = 0.4$ (rad s^{-1}) $D_2 = 1.0$
'Slow' regulation of blood-pressure over elastic behaviour and pressoreceptors of the arterial system	(8.12)	$F_{affl} = \dfrac{\tau_c \cdot p}{1 + \tau_c p} P + K_2(P - P_0)$	F_{affl} = Afferent impulses from pressoreceptors $K_2 = 0.5$ $\tau_c = 0.2$ (s) P = Arterial pressure $P_0 = 40$ (mm Hg)
Heart-rate regulation by vasomotor centre and sinus node	(8.13)	$HR = PF_0 \left(1 - \dfrac{F_{veff}}{a + bF_{veff}}\right)$ $(1 + F_{seffo} + K_{PF}W_s) \left(\dfrac{\omega_{n1}2}{p^2 + 2D_1\omega_{n1}p + \omega_{n1}^2}\right)$	HR = Heart-rate HR_0 = Basic heart-rate without vagal and sympathetic activity F_{veff} = Efferent vagal activity F_{seffo} = Efferent sympathetic activity in rest W_s = Reference variable of sympathico-tonic activity under workload

Such theoretical control and autorhythmic effects of generation of respiration are considered in the model (Koepchen and Baumgarten 1960; Koepchen 1972; Baumgarten, Bolthasar, and Koepchen 1960; Hartung 1966).

Respiration affects blood-pressure by the intrathoracic pressure (eqns (8.6), (8.7), (8.8)) and mechanical coupling (Piiper 1972; Golenhofen and Hildebrandt 1958, 1961; Koepchen 1962a, b). As shown by Miyawaki, Takahashi, and Takemura (1966), respiration is coupled with the pneumatic intrathoracic pressure over a DT_1 transfer function; that means that only changes in pressure result in a disturbance variable (Clynes 1960a, b, c).

Under physical workload, the frequency and amplitude of respiration increase, mostly stimulated by chemical signals. The influence of biochemical and thermal variables on heart-rate variability is neglected in this model, since transfer functions and morphological equivalence with real physiological processes are involved. For this reason the parameters of stimulation of respiration were introduced into the model by approximating the measurements of Hollmann (1959, 1963) for steady-state frequency and amplitude of respiration under physical workload over a function generator. The transit response was matched using data from Piiper (1972) (see eqns (8.9) and (8.10)).

The control of blood-pressure is performed by two separate loops. Their regulating units, peripheral resistance and blood-volume per minute, are connected by a multiplier. The loops can be divided into a 'quick' part—regulating unit 'cardiac output'—and a 'slow' part—regulating unit 'peripheral resistance'. Pressoreceptors and receptors of the vasomotor system serve as sensors in the control loops of blood-pressure. They signal the instantaneous value of blood-pressure to the vasomotor centre. From here, by sympathetic and vagus pathways, the activity of the heart is affected and the peripheral resistance of blood flow is adjusted by the status of contraction of the vascular muscles (Wagner 1954; Koepchen 1962b; Weidinger and Leschhorn 1964; Stegemann and Müller-Bütow 1966; Stegemann and Geisen 1966a, b; Stegemann, Gotke, and Geisen 1966; Hildebrandt 1967; Sayers 1973). The PT_2-transfer function in eqn (8.11) describes the elastic behaviour of the arterial system.

The loops for blood-pressure control are closed over the pressoreceptors and the vasomotor receptors. Their behaviour is described in eqns (8.11), (8.12), and (8.14) (after Miyawaki et al. 1966).

In the vasomotor centre the afferent impulses of the pressoreceptors are transformed into efferent signals influencing the sinus node. The instantaneous value of heart-rate is stimulated by the sinus node, which can be seen as the arithmetic unit combining the effect of several sympathetic and vagal pathways (Miyawaki *et al.* 1966). The oscillatory behaviour of the sinus node is realized in the PT_2-transfer function in eqn (8.13).

Instantaneous heart-rate multiplied by systolic discharge volume leads to a value for blood-volume per minute. With this relation the 'quick' control loop of blood-pressure is fed back over the vasomotor receptors. The afferent impulses of these receptors affect the vasomotor centre and from there influence vascular nerves, vascular muscles, and thus peripheral resistance (see eqns (8.12), (8.14), and (8.15)). The parameters of the system of equations were adjusted in such a manner that, under rest conditions 25 per cent of the output quantity is controlled by the respective loop according to the experimental results of Stegemann and Geisen (1966b).

The relation between peripheral resistance, status of contraction of the vascular muscles, and oxygen requirement (or the physical workload) is a hyperbolic function (after Grimby, Nilson, and Saltin 1966). The decrease of peripheral resistance under the influence of physical workload is detected by receptors in the muscles according to the results of Stegemann (1971). By adjusting the effect of the muscle receptors on sympathetic pathways and on peripheral resistance the behaviour of heart-rate under physical stress and the relation between blood-pressure and heart-rate could be adjusted.

The rhythm of blood-pressure is generated by rhythmic variations of vasomotor tone, which are treated as autorhythmic fluctuations either within the vasomotor centre or within a higher centre of the nervous system (eqns (8.17) and (8.18)). In the model this is simulated by a sinusoidal oscillator which is synchronized in amplitude and frequency by the vasomotor receptors. When the respective receptors are cut off, the blood-pressure variations decrease in amplitude and frequency according to Weidinger and Leschhorn (1964), Wagner (1954), and Koepchen (1962a).

Under physical workload the increase of heart-rate is controlled by sympathetic tone. The stimuli are generated within receptors in the muscle. The effects of these stimuli are described by a model developed by Brodan, Hajek, and Kuhn (1971). This model was used partially with modifications where the reaction of heart-rate below the endurance limit (aerobic work) was concerned (eqns (8.19), (8.20), (8.21), (8.22)).

Simulation runs

For the simulation runs a Telefunken RA 800 analogue computer was used and the results were plotted by a six-channel Beckman plotter. Figs 8.2 and 8.3 show simulation runs with a step function of physical workload with 50- and 200-W ergometer work. The endurance limit of the model reaction was set to 100 W. The model shows the characteristic increase of heart-rate below and beyond the endurance limit and the superimposition of a quick and a slow component of decrease during the phase of recovery following anaerobic work. Mean arterial pressure, peripheral resistance, and respiratory activity show the expected behaviour which is documented in the literature. The rhythmic interactions cause a fluctuation in heart-rate, i.e. they are the *deterministic components* of heart-rate variability. With increasing physical workload and increasing heart rate, HRV decreases according to the results of Laurig *et al.* (1971); (see Fig. 8.4).

The relation between blood-pressure (mean arterial pressure) and heart-rate is given in Fig. 8.5. The model results show a similar trend though at a slightly different level, to those of the measurements of Holmgren (1956) and Stegemann (1971).

Varying the physical workload sinusoidally in frequency between 0 and 0·1 Hz and in amplitude between 8 and 80 W according to the experimental conditions of Stegemann (1963) results in the amplitude and phase-angle response shown in Fig. 8.6. Experimental results and simulation show congruent behaviour.

The increase of heart-rate under non-physical workload—as measured by the number of decisions per minute taken in a binary choice task (Kalsbeek 1967)—is followed in principle by the model: dynamically in the transient response (Fig. 8.7 and Coles 1972), and in the steady-state with respect to the results of Laurig and Philipp (1970) and Ettema and Zielhuis (1971); see Fig. 8.8. The time-dependent behaviour of several physiological parameters under non-physical stress is shown in Fig. 8.9. The decrease of HRV and increase of blood-pressure and frequency of respiration can be clearly distinguished. Simulation runs to examine respiratory arrhythmia show results congruent with the experimental findings of Angelone and Coulter (1964).

Discussion

The purpose of the model is to explain the basic physiological variations of instantaneous heart-rate with the help of control theory and

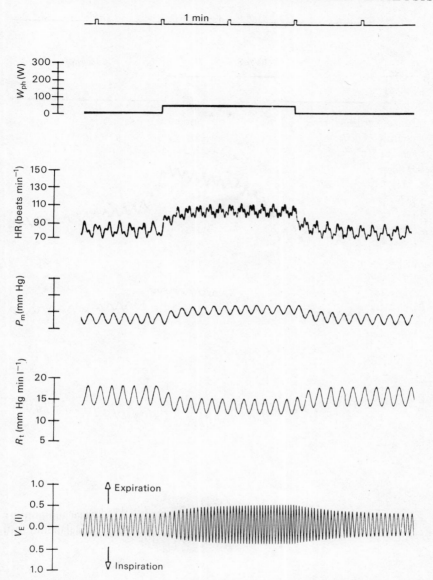

F$_{\text{IG}}$. 8.2. Transient response of model parameters—instantaneous heart-rate (HR), mean arterial pressure (P_m), peripheral resistance (R_t), ventilation (V_E)—after a step function of physical workload—50 W aerobic ergometer work.

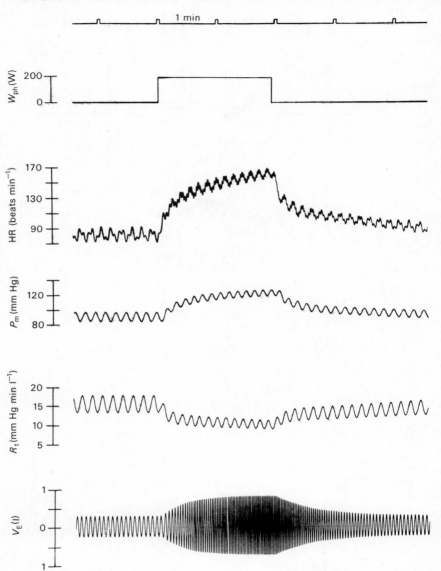

FIG. 8.3. Transient response of model parameters—instantaneous heart-rate (HR), mean arterial pressure (P_m), peripheral resistance (R_t), ventilation (V_E)—after a step function of physical workload—200 W anaerobic ergometer work.

136

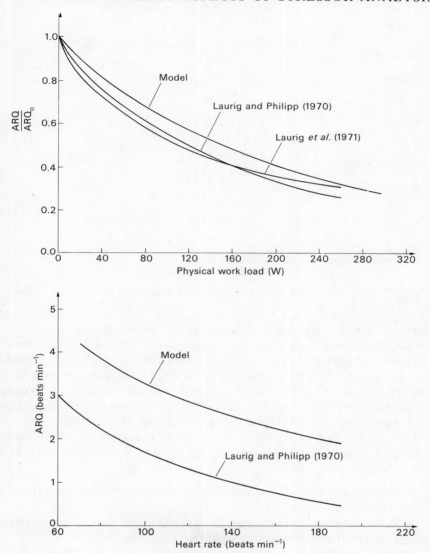

FIG. 8.4. Heart-rate variability, scored by ARQ, in relation to physical workload and heart-rate.

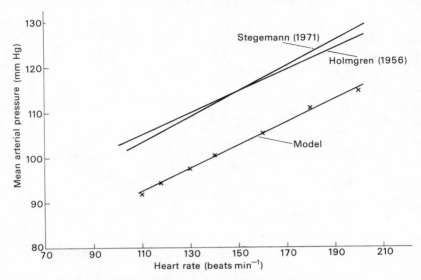

FIG. 8.5. Relation between blood-pressure and heart-rate.

systems analysis. The models of the human cardiovascular and cardio-respiratory control system previously presented have mostly considered the 'low'-frequency variations of mean heart-rate (Pickering, Nikiforuk, and Merriman 1969) or specific aspects of the 'high'-frequency variations, for instance some reflexes like the carotid sinus reflex (Scher and Young 1963; Levison, Barnett, and Jackson 1966) or the coupling of respiration and heart-rate (Clynes 1960a, b, c; Miyawaki et al. 1966; Womack 1971). In the system described here the superimposition of the most important effects on HRV in a frequency band from 0·005 to 0·5 Hz in a single model is demonstrated:

> frequency and depth of respiration with central and reflex generation of the respiratory functions;
> blood-pressure variations due to autorhythmic and control-system effects, coupled with the vasomotor tone;
> effects of physical work load on all physiological functions considered—aerobic and anaerobic work and the appropriate phases of recovery.

Temperature variation is assumed to influence HRV, but is neglected in the model because the implications concern a frequency band which does not severely affect scores of HRV under mental load.

138

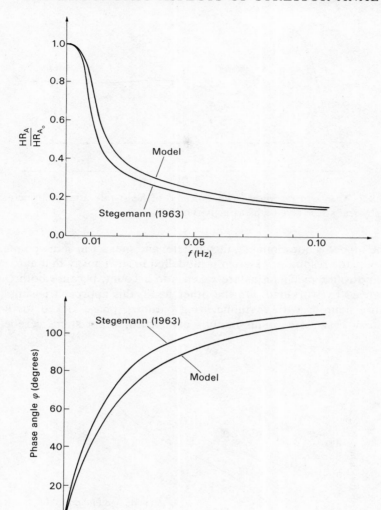

FIG. 8.6. Amplitude and phase angle response curve on sinusoidally changed physical workload (8–80 W; 0–0·1 Hz).

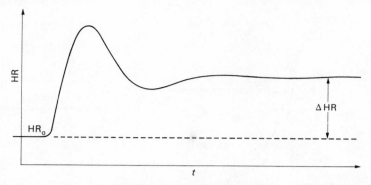

FIG. 8.7. Transient response (schematically) of heart-rate after step increase of non-physical stress (sympathicus activity).

The model is questionable, incomplete, and inexact in some points. For instance, the respiratory system is modelled in such a way that autorhythmic and reflex mechanisms are taken into account, because both can be influenced by workload. On the other hand, this approach is simplified, because neurons with rhythmic firing patterns, phase-locked to the respiratory cycle, are found in the spinal cord, brain stem, cerebellum,

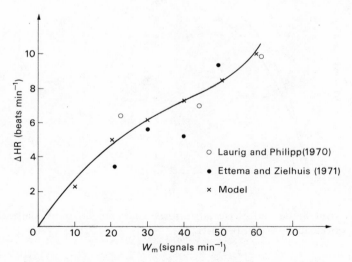

FIG. 8.8. Increase of heart-rate as a function of mental load.

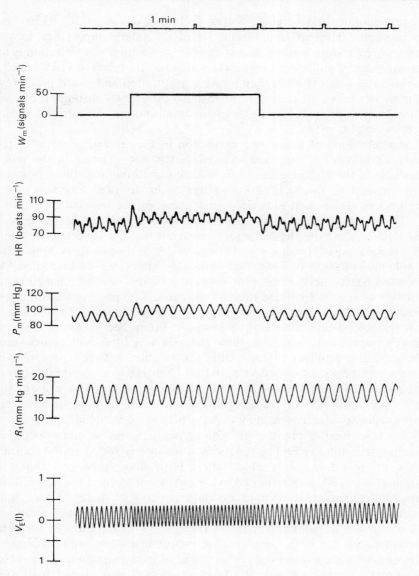

FIG. 8.9. Transient response of model parameters—instantaneous heart-rate (HR), mean arterial pressure (P_m), peripheral resistance (R_t), ventilation (V_E)—after a step function of non-physical stress—sympathicus activity.

141

hypothalamus, and cerebral cortex (Feldman and Cowan 1975b), and because the Hering–Breuer reflex is of secondary importance for the human respiratory system. The system for generation of respiration is too complex to be modelled adequately within the approach to HRV which is considered here. The coupling between respiration and blood-pressure in the model takes account only of mechanical aspects through the transmural aortic pressure, though experimental findings indicate that neural pathways also exist.

An inhibition of vasomotor oscillation in the arterial pressure system under workload is supposed to exist, but is not included in the model because of the lack of quantitative description. Some simplifications must be ascribed to the lack of knowledge about transfer functions of the respective system and to limited analogue computer capacity.

The model provides some insights for the interpretation of the decrease of HRV under non-physical stress, though it was not especially designed for this purpose. Hyndman and Gregory (1975) discuss three hypotheses explaining changes of heart-rate variability under mental load: first 'decreased heart-rate baroreceptor-reflex sensitivity'; second 'change in the pattern of respiration'; and third 'change in the frequency of spontaneous vasomotor oscillations by changes in the time delay in the feedback loop of the blood-pressure control system'. From the point of view of psychophysiological research, these theories have little explanatory value, because the problem of explaining the relation between psychological cause and physiological effect is shifted from HRV to another, inferred, physiological function. Nevertheless the model presented here shows that all these above-mentioned mechanisms within the cardiorespiratory and the cardiovascular system may depress heart-rate variability.

In this model mental or non-physical stress is introduced by sympathetic-tone reference functions. Its value is added to the 'normal' flow of neural impulses which affect both sinus node and centre of respiration. HRV is determined to a great extent by the above-mentioned rhythmic variables; the amplitude and frequency of these rhythmic variables are influenced by the activity of vagus and sympathetic pathways. An increase in neural activity is thought to affect transfer elements non-linearly, as for the amplification factors in the physiological control circuits, which are dependent on the level of parasympathetic tone, which is directly connected with the level of arousal and mental load. The saturation characteristic of the transfer elements causes a relatively decreased output function with linearly increased input function; this means, physiologically, a depression of HRV. Thus it can be supposed that the amplitude of the autonomous centrally induced, respiratory, vasomotor, and sinus-node rhythms is reduced by co-innervation, in the sense of a disturbance-variable, feed-forward system. Entrainment effects (Sayers 1973) between the various rhythmic systems and their non-linear superimposition can cause additional depression in the amplitude and frequency response of instantaneous heart-rate to workload.

8.4. Experiments on superimposition of components of stress

In the model of HRV the effect of non-physical stress, i.e. mental load produced by a definite task and the emotional basis of arousal, was introduced by vagal and sympathetic activity in the form of a reference function. From the point of view of psychophysiological research it seems unsatisfactory and oversimplified to have only one neural pathway to connect the parasympathetic with the somatic nervous system, i.e. ergonomically one type of stress–strain interaction.

The purpose of the experiments to be described was to assess different types of strain with relation to their effect on HRV.

Scoring heart-rate variability

In the experiments instantaneous heart-rate was measured by recording the ECG telemetrically, determining RR intervals by an electronic timer, and storing the data sequentially on a magnetic tape or disc. In the computer the HRV was scored by calculating a measure of it, the ARQ, according to the method given by Laurig *et al.* (1971) (see Fig. 8.10):

$$ARQ = \frac{\sum_{i=1}^{n-1} (HR_i - HR_{i+1}) \forall_i : (HR_i - HR_{i+1}) > 0}{H_n[\{(HR_i > HR_{i+1}) \wedge (HR_i > HR_{i-1})\} \\ \vee \{(HR_i < HR_{i+1}) \wedge (HR_i < HR_{i-1})\}]} \; min^{-1},$$

where n is the interval of registration of heart-rate or the number of beat-to-beat registrations; i is the running index; HR_i is the measured value of instantaneous heart-rate at index point i; $\forall_i$ is all elements i; and H_n is the frequency of events in the interval n.

The ARQ contains amplitude information in the numerator and frequency information in the denominator. In the numerator the sum of the beat-to-beat differences within a given interval n is calculated for all

143

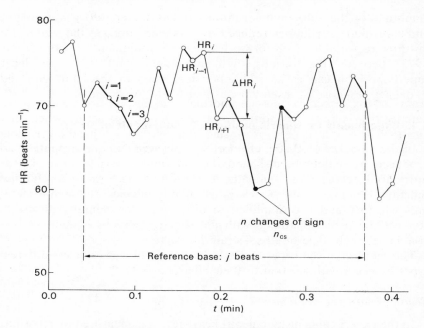

FIG. 8.10. Basic parameters of HRV and their derivation.

cases, when heart-rate is decreasing from beat to beat. For a steady state of the heart-rate time series, the sum of beat-to-beat differences with increasing heart-rate must be approximately the same within the limits of the measurement technique.

With the comparison of positive and negative sums of interbeat interval differences, the criterion of steady-state is checked. After this check the respective sum can be taken as numerator. It has the dimension beats min^{-1} like heart-rate. In the denominator the frequency of relative maxima and minima in the time series heart-rate within a given interval is identified. This number has no physical dimension. The quotient ARQ therefore has the dimension min^{-1}. It is something like a mean value of amplitude, namely the mean value of all spans between interbeat intervals with changing direction of fluctuation.

The performance data of information-processing were transformed into information flows with the known algorithms of information theory (Attneave 1968) to have a comparable scale of information load.

Experiment 1: *Stress by a binary choice reaction task with increased signal rate combined with movements of hands, arms, and upper part of the body*

Problem. This experiment is concerned with the influence of motor actions, superimposed on a mental task, on heart-rate variability. The physical stress of these motor actions was set far below the endurance limits of the respective muscles and the cardiorespiratory system. It was intended to simulate conditions, as they normally occur, when in a practical task information-processing and information-handling is done with motor actions leading to information perception and output.

Method. The apparatus used was a binary choice generator similar to that of Kalsbeek (1967), which in a modified form presents two different visual signals to the subject, which have to be answered on a keyboard. In a first session the signal rate was set to 0 (rest), 20 (endurance limit according to Kalsbeek 1967), 40, and 60 signals per minute (minimal interindividual maximum according to Kalsbeek 1967) with no motor action except for handling the keyboard. In a second experimental session 0, 30, and 50 signals per minute were presented combined with an additional 10 defined movements per minute of the hand (5 cm), hand + arm (30 cm), hand + arm + upper part of the body (60 cm). The decision task was connected with the motor actions in a 3^2-factorial experimental design. The experiments lasted 4 min each and were interrupted by pauses of 4 min.

The experimental conditions within the sessions were permutated arbitrarily. Forty-eight male subjects were used of mean age 26·5 years, SD 6·7; mean height 180·1 cm, SD 5·7; mean weight 71·9 kg, SD 7·3; all were students or personnel of the institute.

Results and interpretation. The results of the first session (18 subjects) are shown in relation to those of the second (30 subjects) in Fig. 8.11. The variation of the measurements on the abscissa (flow of transinformation) is caused by different fault rates and changes in the homogeneous presentation of the signals, in addition to the experimental effect. In the measurements scaled on the ordinate two main influences can be distinguished: under experimental conditions without any disturbances by motor actions, the level of heart-rate variability is lower and the correlation to information-processing is higher than in the experimental conditions with motor actions. Hence measurements of heart-rate variability for the purpose of evaluation of mental strain are considerably distorted by the effects of motor actions.

145

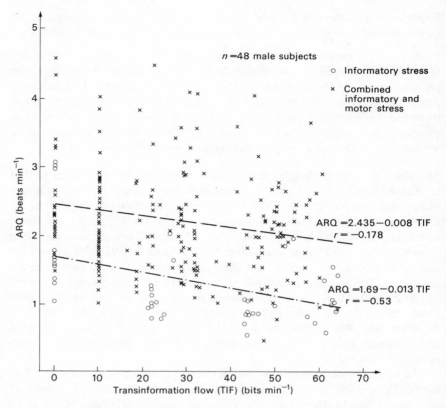

FIG. 8.11. Scored heart-rate variability (ARQ) as a function of mental load (task speed) and motor actions.

A two-way analysis of variance with interactions applied to the data of the first session shows that the interindividual variance is of the same magnitude as the intraindividual variance caused by the experimental conditions (Table 8.2). The interaction between subjects and stress is still significant. From these results it can be concluded that each subject has a specific level of HRV, the pattern of which is subject-dependent and should be eliminated by appropriate corrections. The results of the second session could be further analysed as to the effect of different stresses on HRV because of the factorial experimental design. A correlation analysis was calculated between all relevant influences on HRV.

146

TABLE 8.2

Analysis of variance of measurements of heart-rate variability

	Variance	Degrees of freedom	F-Test	α
Subjects	5·067	17	25·47	0·01
Stress	5·814	3	29·23	0·001
Interaction	0·815	9	4·10	0·05
Rest variance	0·199	216	—	—

Hypothetically the value of an ARQ can be determined by the function

$$ARQ = f(HR; W_{mot}; W_{ment}; W_{emot}; ITG),$$

where HR is the level of heart-rate, W_{mot} is the motor part of strain, W_{ment} is the mental part of strain, W_{emot} is the emotional part of strain, and ITG represents the individual traits and capacities of the subject. The correlation analysis was restricted to these variables. A direct measurement of emotional stress is not available in the experimental design. Proceeding from the hypothesis that the novelty of the experimental situation increases the level of activation but that this anticipation stress decreases with the number of sessions in the experiment, the consecutive number of sessions was taken as a parameter of emotional stress.

An operable normalization for the individual physiological response seems to be the 'range correction', proposed by Lykken (1972),

$$HR_N = \frac{HR - HR_{min}}{HR_{max} - HR_{min}} \qquad ARQ_N = \frac{ARQ - ARQ_{min}}{ARQ_{max} - ARQ_{min}}.$$

This 'range correction' eliminates individual differences in level and tendency of reaction of a measured variable. It seems to be a better normalization than the relation of the measurements to a rest value which is usually used, because mental rest conditions cannot be controlled and such conditions have the greatest intraindividual variance. The results of the correlation analysis with and without 'range correction' are given in Table 8.3. The correlations of the hypothetical relations are weak but partially significant ($R_{crit,0·05} = 0·13$). The highest correlation exists between heart-rate and motor actions, as expected, but the other correlations between ARQ and HR and ARQ and mental load are significant too. With the range correction the correlations in the direction of the

TABLE 8.3

Correlations between different types of stress and heart-rate variability (ARQ)/heart-rate (HR)

	With original measurements				With normalized values after 'range correction'			
	HR	W_{mot}	W_{ment}	W_{emot}	HR	W_{mot}	W_{ment}	W_{emot}
ARQ	−0·18	−0·069	−0·178	−0·018	−0·124	−0·099	−0·296	−0·041
HR		0·232	0·091	0·12		0·604	0·137	0·101

experimental effect increase considerably. The intraindividual mean values of the experimental conditions were taken as basic values for the range correction.

If the variation of the measurements in the direction of the experimental effect is maximal, the range correction really is an appropriate method to increase correlation and thus to get results which can be interpreted more easily. The table of correlations shows that the level of heart-rate and HRV are coupled. To test the hypothesis that HRV does not contain any information about mental strain, if heart-rate is kept constant, a partial correlation between HRV and mental strain with constant heart-rate was calculated. The resulting correlation coefficient was −0·284 and indicated that the hypothesis must be rejected, i.e. under these experimental conditions HRV actually contains additional information for the assessment of strain.

Experiment 2: Stress by a multiple-choice reaction task with increased task difficulty

Problem. This experiment is concerned with the influence of information transmission, varied by task difficulty, and of emotional tension on heart-rate variability. The experiments with the binary choice generator include with increasing mental load an increase in motor actions, because the signal reaction rate per unit time is varied. Possibly the whole physiological reaction must be attributed to the motor reactions (Danev, Wartna, and Radder 1971); this hypothesis can be tested, if experimental conditions are chosen which vary information transmission by different task difficulty at constant speed.

Method. The apparatus used was a multiple-choice reaction generator, built with a Massey–Dickenson system. The subjects had to fulfil a forced choice-reaction task with 2, 4, 6, 8, 9 choice-reaction alternatives, which had to be answered in 1·4 s each. The experimental conditions followed one another in a 5 min work–rest schedule. To assess emotional and mental strain in one diagram, the task difficulty was increased regularly with the consecutive number of sessions (see measurement of emotional stress in experiment 1). Twenty female subjects were used of mean age 37·7 years, SD 9; mean height 163·2 cm, SD 7·9, mean weight 65·2 kg, SD 7·0; all personnel who were highly skilled in various typing tasks.

Results and interpretation. Because of the specific design of the experimental procedure, different types of strain could be separated in Fig. 8.12. On the ordinate the measurements of heart-rate (Fig. 8.12(a)) and heart-rate variability (Fig. 8.12(b)) respectively are shown. On the abscissa two scales are available, one representing an increasing mental load measured by input information rate, the other representing a decreasing emotional stress measured by the novelty of the experimental situation in terms of 5-min phases.

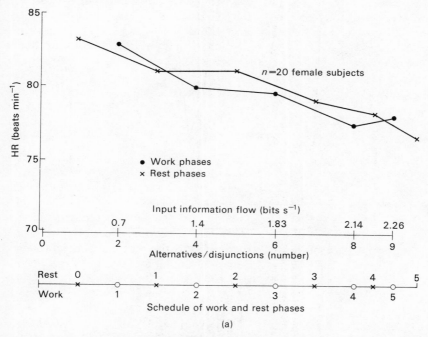

(a)

FIG. 8.12. (a) Heart-rate and (b) scored heart-rate variability (ARQ) as functions of mental load (task difficulty) and the series of experimental sessions.

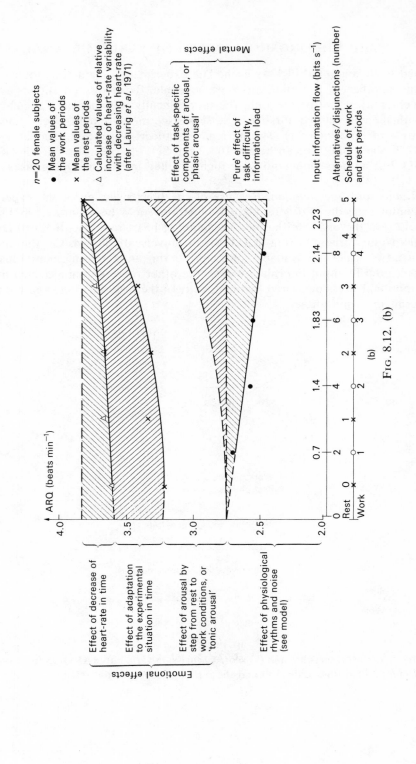

FIG. 8.12. (b)

Heart-rate decreases significantly as a function of the duration of the experiment and is independent of task difficulty. There is not even a significant difference between the interindividual means of all work and rest phases. It thus appears that the often-measured increase of heart-rate under mental load conditions documented in the literature, can be attributed either to a simultaneous increase of motor actions or to an emotional strain, which could not be clearly separated from the mental load owing to the design of the particular experiment.

HRV decreases interindividually with increasing difficulty of the task; i.e. the hypothesis can be rejected that the whole reaction of HRV in information load tasks is due to increased motor activity. The measurements of HRV in the rest phases increase with the duration of the experiment. This is partly due to the decrease of heart-rate. This can be evaluated quantitatively by considering the results of experiments on the relation between the level of heart-rate and heart-rate variability scored by ARQ (see Fig. 8.13). The results were obtained from a group of 30 male subjects, mean age 27·1 years, SD 5·7; mean height 178·5 cm, SD 7·1; mean weight 74·4 kg, SD 8·5; in bicycle ergometer activities (workload 5 to 250 W at 60 rev/min duration of each load phase 5–15 min).

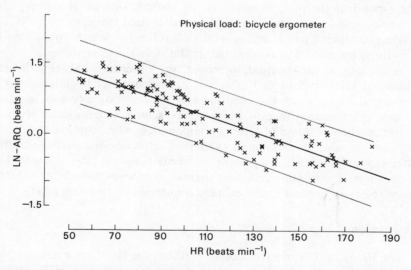

FIG. 8.13. Functional relationship between heart-rate variability (ARQ) and heart-rate (HR); logarithmic transformation of ARQ and linear regression line with 95 per cent prediction limits.

Applying this knowledge of the quantitative relation between heart-rate and HRV to the respective values of HRV in the experiment on mental task difficulty, a first component of HRV can be removed from the whole experimental effect. But, as shown in Fig. 8.13, only a small part of the time-dependent increase of HRV in the rest periods can be explained by this effect. Using the concept of different specifications of arousal, however (e.g. Lindsley 1961 with his separation of 'common' and 'local' arousal, and Sharpless and Jasper 1956 discussing 'tonic' and 'phasic' arousal), we can conclude that there is a component of arousal, produced by task difficulty, which can be called phasic arousal, because it varies rather quickly with the phases of external workload (see also §8.5).

The remaining part of the time-dependent increase of HRV in the rest periods can be attributed to different types of strain by a hypothetical model of components of strain. According to the 'information load model' HRV should decrease with increased information-processing. Therefore a purely information-dependent component of strain was separated from the whole reaction by extrapolating the regression line $HRV = f$ (information load) to a fictive information-processing of 0 bit s^{-1}.

According to the 'arousal model' a certain level of arousal is necessary to perform a task. This level of arousal has a constant component that corresponds to the jump from rest to work conditions, because every kind of performance requests a certain level of arousal (tonic arousal). It also has a component which varies with task difficulty, which could also be explained by the 'information load model' (phasic arousal).

According to the 'adaptation model' the difference between the rest values of HRV before and after the experiment can be interpreted as emotional strain, which is decreasing with the adaptation to and 'learning' of the experimental situation, which can be seen as a stress factor itself.

In the whole reaction of HRV a component can be distinguished, which is due to the experimental situation—situation-induced emotional components—and a component, that is due to the information-processing—information-induced mental components—which together form the non-physical strain expressed in terms of variation of HRV.

Discusssion

The problems of different scoring methods for HRV are excluded from the discussion. Nearly all investigators doing research in HRV 'found' their individual 'best' scores that deliver quantitatively incomparable results between different publications. On the other hand, all scores presented are variability scores showing the same tendency and using the same information parameters, namely frequency and/or amplitude characteristics in the series of values of instantaneous heart-rate. The experimental results show that HRV is a physiological variable, which is affected by almost every imaginable ergonomic influence. It is correlated with the level of heart-rate (see also Laurig *et al.* 1971; Rohmert 1973; Mulder and Mulder-Hajonides 1973; Blitz, Hoogstraten, and Mulder (1970), and therefore it depends on physical workload (Clynes 1960*a*, *b*; Laurig and Philipp 1970; Laurig *et al.* 1971; Rohmert *et al.* 1973). Even small motor actions, which should not have measurable effects on the metabolic rate, influence HRV over neutral pathways. Similar results were found by Mulder and Mulder-Hajonides (1973). They show a characteristic maximum in the spectrum of HRV at the frequency of a tapping task and confirm our results. From the point of view of psychic stress, the mental load and spare mental capacity model (Kalsbeek 1967; Ettema 1967; Wartna, Danev, and Bink 1971) as well as the arousal and activation model (Zwaga 1973; Porges and Raskin 1969; Porges 1972) can be used to interpret the experimental results. Therefore the model of components of HRV was developed which gives room for both. The mental load model cannot explain the effect of time on task reported here (see also Strasser 1974 and Gaillard and Trumbo 1976), whereas the arousal and activation concept is unable to explain the slight and approximately linear decrease of HRV with speed and difficulty of the experimental task. The step in scores of HRV from rest to work conditions (see also Hyndman and Gregory 1975) can be assigned to a 'jump' in arousal more than to the relatively low mental load in the easiest experimental condition.

In addition HRV is influenced by drugs (Strasser 1974; Gaillard and Trumbo 1976), physiological functions like respiration, blood pressure, and other rhythmic variables (see the theoretical control model and Clynes 1960*a*, *b*), and individual variables such as age and sex (Malmö and Shagass 1949). The complexity of the influences on HRV makes it extremely difficult to interpret changes in HRV measured under field situations (Rohmert *et al.* 1973). The effect measured cannot be attributed to a specific postulated influence, because it can be masked by many other influences, which are superimposed on the 'expected' variation of HRV. A more detailed investigation of HRV can be done, however, if the complexity of the influences is taken into account by simultaneous registration of different physiological variables and cross-analysis of their reaction.

8.5. Polygraphic assessment of physiological indicators of arousal

A third approach to the evaluation of heart-rate variability, using a concept of polygraphic measurement of physiological reactions, is based on the psychophysiological concept of arousal or activation. This concept is characterized by the hypothesis of a functional entity of awareness of stress, behavioural activities, and physiological reactions which are controlled by a central regulating process (Duffy 1957). The consequence of this central process is a variation of the cortical arousal level (Lindsley 1960). This cortical activity which is necessary for a specific information-processing task of a human operator is steered by subcortical structures of the reticular formation and of the limbic system (Haider 1969). In this process the non-specific influence of sensory impulses on the reticular formation plays an important role in determining the level of arousal (Lynn 1966). Simultaneously, the information perceived is assessed by the limbic system with respect to emotional reactions and thus provides an additional influence on the level of arousal (Routtenberg 1968). Haider (1969) assigns a hierarchical system of states of arousal to the neuro-psychological mechanisms mentioned earlier. His concept implies research results on components of arousal found by Lindsley (1961), Sokolow (1963), and Sharpless and Jasper (1956). Four levels of arousal are described: first regulation of sleep and wakefulness; second a generalized state of arousal with only slow fluctuations of the arousal level, called 'tonic' arousal; third quick variations of arousal, which can be related to specific physiological systems, which are called 'phasic' arousal; and fourth arousal mechanisms which are selective with respect to discrimination among the natures of external stimuli. The processes of tonic and phasic arousal in particular have an explicative value for the ergonomic investigation of heart-rate variability. Trying to differentiate different states of arousal by physiological reactions, implies a polygraphic measurement concept, which takes into account indicators of central nervous activity as well as peripheral parasympathetic reactions, which can be related to the states of phasic and tonic arousal. As a central nervous indicator of arousal, electroencephalographic (EEG) measurements are discussed in the literature (Lindsley 1960). In the context of analysis of heart-rate variability the cardiorespiratory parameters, heart-rate, and respiration rate, have to be taken into account. The interaction between central nervous activity and peripheral parasympathetic reactions are based not only on neural pathways but also on humoral control mechanisms. Thus the polygraphic concept must be widened to include the registration of the catecholamines, adrenalin and noradrenalin, as important biochemical indicators of arousal (Euler 1964; Friedhoff 1975).

Analysis of single indicators of arousal

Electroencephalogram. The results on using electroencephalographic measurements as indicators of arousal are contradictory. Consequently methodological studies on the differentiation of EEG-parameters with respect to different states of arousal in information workload experiments had to be performed. Spectral analysis of EEG registration in different experiments show that variations of arousal simultaneous to external workload can be expected in specific EEG-frequency bands: for the theta-activity (4–7 Hz) several authors found an increase in amplitude in different situations of non-physical stress (Mundy-Castle 1957; Adey 1969; Bente, Frick, Lewinsky, Penning, and Scheuler 1976). A general increase in amplitude of the beta-activity (15–30 Hz) with respect to mental load in comparison to rest conditions is reported (Glaser 1963; Legewie, Simonova, and Creutzfeld 1970). The results of these authors were verified by our own experiments concerning spectral analysis of EEG during different information workload situations. Taking into account these results and the ergonomic demands of continuous registration over long times and of quantification of parameters as a time series synchronous to other variables, methods other than spectral analysis have to be developed. One method is to filter an appropriate frequency band out of the EEG-signal, rectify it, and the resulting amplitudes are integrated over definite intervals of time. Thus an equidistant series of digital values is achieved, representing the EEG activity in the specific frequency band. The resulting values of this procedure are known as the 'electrical activity' (EA) of an electrophysiological signal, mostly known and applied in electromyographical research (Lippold 1952). To evaluate these EEG-parameters with respect to a differentiation between states of arousal under the conditions of mental load an experiment was performed. The simulation of mental load was done by a multiple-choice reaction task as described in §8.4 (Experiment 2).

Besides varying the difficulty of the task by varying the number of choice-reaction alternatives (ALT), the amount of mental load was also changed by varying the signal rate. Signal rate is calculated as a constant factor of minimal individual reaction time (reaction time factor, RTF). The objective of the experiments was to find the maximal endurance in this information-processing task, under the condition that a constant error ratio of 5 per cent would not be exceeded. In the experiments EEG was recorded bipolarly with surface disc electrodes in the position O_2–P_4 due to the international 10–20 system. Twenty seconds was chosen as the integration-time constant for the calculation of the EA-values.

The results are shown in Fig. 8.14. The presented EEG-values were normalized according to a range correction procedure as described in §4 (Experiment 1). On the left-hand side of Fig. 8.14, the variation of theta- and beta-activity is shown as a function of the normalized duration of the respective trials (T_{max}). The EA-values were calculated as means over the rest period or over intervals of 20 per cent of the normalized duration.

The behaviour of theta-activity is characterized by an initial increase with overshoot in the beginning of the session and a monotonic increase following until the previously defined criterion for the endurance limit is reached. The level of theta-activity is clearly a function of work difficulty, i.e. the number of ALT. This phenomenon occurs even in the rest period before the experimental session, an effect which can be related to expectancy based on beforehand knowledge of the ALT-condition and thus to a situationally induced tonic arousal. The shape of the EA-beta-curve is similar, but no distinction between the ALT-conditions is visible. If the influence of signal rate is taken into account, however, the mean values of EA-beta-activity show a functional relationship to RTF, i.e. time pressure, and even to total mental load quantified by input information flow ($H(x, t)$). Because an increase in input information flow means an increase in the rate of central nervous activity, i.e. the combination of sensory afferent input and motor efferent output, beta-activity can be interpreted as an indicator of task-specific phasic arousal.

Catecholamines. The quick and selective adjustment of organic functions to the presence of stressors is guaranteed by neural control. The common and persistent adaptation toward a sympathetic activation of all areas of the parasympathetic nervous system is done by increased excretion of catecholamines from the adrenal medulla into the bloodstream (Keidel 1973; Bechtereva, Kamborova, and Pozdeev 1975; Randall 1977). Catecholamine production is controlled by neural pathways from the central nervous system. Besides higher structures, areas of the hypothalamus are involved predominantly. In the hypothalamus many afferent and efferent connections from and to the forebrain and brainstem constitute the network which involves this area in high level integrations between somatic, autonomic, and endocrine functions (Caspers 1973; Sigg 1975).

An analysis of the literature shows that the measured increase of catecholamine secretion under psychic load is caused primarily by an

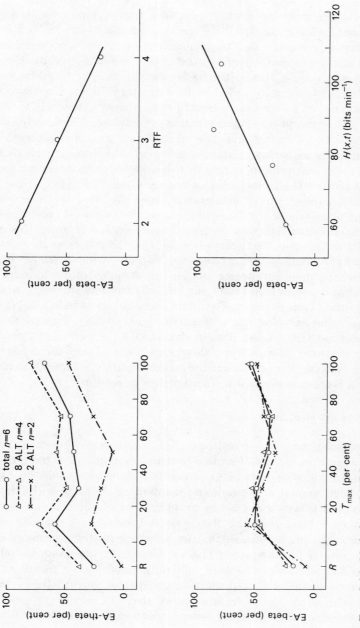

Fig. 8.14. Variation of EEG theta- and beta-activity at different numbers of choice reaction alternatives (ALT) as a function of normalized experimental time (T_{max}), reaction time factor (RTF), and signal input information flow ($H(x, t)$); rest phase (R); for further information refer to text.

increase of adrenalin secretion and, to a minor extent, by noradrenalin secretion. Different authors conclude that this has to be seen as a result of a common activation and as an indicator of the psychophysically perceived emotional component of stress (Hale, Williams, and Buckley 1969; Hoagland, Bergen, Bloch, Elmadjian, and Gibree 1955; Mason 1971; Levi 1972; Mandler 1967; Pekkarinen, Castren, Iisalo, Koivusalo, Laihinen, Simola, and Thomasson 1961; Frankenhäuser 1969, 1975). According to a concept of differentiation of different levels of arousal, catecholamine secretion indicates a preparation of the organism in the face of expected stressor situations, that is, the first step in a chain of consecutive reactions to stress. In this context, catecholamine secretion can be interpreted as indicator of tonic arousal.

Catecholamines can be determined in the plasma or by their excretion into the urine (Euler 1964). For ergonomic investigations only the assessment from an analysis of the urinary excretion is tolerable. This method restricts the insight into the emotionally effected processes to a successive evaluation by data sampling over long periods—urine collection intervals. In the experiments reported above the samples of urine were taken before the beginning and after the end of the stress situation, which will be explained later in detail. To obtain control data as individual reference values, urine samples were taken on several days without the stress situation but at the same time of day as in the experimental conditions. The collection intervals were about two hours. To eliminate deviations among collection intervals, and differences in urine volumes, the results of analysis were transformed to the dimensions $ng\,min^{-1}$.

Analysis of interactions

Stressor situation. To investigate the interactions between different physiological indicators of arousal, a stressor situation has to be chosen in which considerable physiological reaction dynamics could be expected and a high mental and emotional component of stress with continuous information-processing could be presumed. In addition it is advantageous to choose a task, in which the subjects involved are familiar with the measurement procedure, so that its influence on the emotional component of stress is minimized. That is why university examinations were chosen as the model task and individuals were taken as subjects who performed a diploma or doctoral thesis in the Institut für Arbeitswissenschaft.

A survey of the literature with respect to different tasks which are

158

combined with considerable amounts of mental and emotional strain (Table 8.4), shows that university examinations lie in the upper part of heart-rate dynamics in comparison to a number of different information-processing tasks with additional emotional components, such as aeroplane piloting, parachute jumping, vehicle driving, operating and control tasks, the tasks of surgeons, musicians, and conductors. (Table 8.4 can also be seen as a survey of non-physical tasks, in which the low-frequency range of heart-rate variability is mentioned.

The examinations are held in oral form. They begin with a report on the thesis (lecture) which is followed by a discussion between the candidate and the audience about the results presented. This part is followed by an oral examination by the professor, which ends with the information about the mark achieved. This whole procedure is called a 'colloquium'. As a control for the individual dynamics of physiological reactions, a phase with a standardized stressor situation before and after the experimental phase was introduced. For this purpose a mental arithmetic test which lasted 10 min each time was chosen (Arnold 1961). Five male subjects with mean age 26 years were involved in the experiments.

Measurement techniques. The recording of ECG and EEG, of the derived indicators HR, ARQ, and EA-EEG, and the collection of urine samples for the determination of catecholamines was done according to the methods described above. The task requires that the ability to speak must not be restricted. Thus, only the frequency of respiration could be registered with the help of a nasal thermistor. All data which were recorded continuously were transmitted by radio telemetry.

Results. In 8.15 the time behaviour of the different indicators for one of the experiments is shown. The plotted values are means over 1 min. For this diagram the signal measurements were normalized with respect to the mean value of the control period, that is the mental arithmetic test phase after the end of the colloquium:

$$y_n(t) = \frac{y_i(t) - \bar{y}}{\bar{y}} \cdot 100 \text{ per cent,}$$

where $y_n(t)$ is the normalized value at sampling time t, $y_i(t)$ is the absolute value at sampling time t, and $\bar{y}$ is the mean value of the control period. By this procedure different directions of deviation are treated equally and the dynamics of the deviation is scaled without dimension.

TABLE 8.4

A collection of some results from a literature survey concerning heart-rate dynamics during different non-laboratory tasks with a predominantly mental and emotional load

Reference	Description of activity	Heart-rate reaction		Comment
		Absolute value (beats min⁻¹)	Increase (beats min⁻¹ or per cent)	

Reference	Description of activity	Absolute value (beats min⁻¹)	Increase (beats min⁻¹ or per cent)	Comment
	Aeroplane pilots			
Rowen 1961	X-15	160		During end of acceleration stage and landing
Howitt, Balkwill, Whiteside, and Whittingsham 1965	Civil			
Roman 1965	Jet fighter			Above rest values: during preparation for and execution of landing and take-off
Smith 1967	Civil		30–50	
Kötz 1968	Helicopter			
Nicholson, Hill, Borland, and Ferres 1970	Civil		40 per cent	Mission for the control of forest fire
Balke, Melton, and Blake 1966	Civil		100 per cent	Emergency training (auto-rotation)
Hoffman, Strubel, Raabe, and Koch 1969	Helicopter			During stunt flying
Eichler and Lobsien 1970	motor-/sail-plane	125		
	Parachute jumping			
Renemann, Beckhove, and Roskamm 1968	Trainees	up to 220		Before and during unfolding of the parachute
Reid and Doerr 1970	Trainees			
Shane and Slinde 1968	Experts	100		

Reference	Activity	Heart rate (beats/min)	Increase	Condition
	Vehicle driving			
Broicher and Dupuis 1963	Automobile		30–40	During passing or heavy traffic
Rapp, Dietlein, and Nuttall 1965	Racing car	120–65		Max. values during start
Sadowski 1976	Train	100		Entrance into or passing a station
Kiczak and Czyzewska 1976	Train	140		Sudden braking
Rohmert and Rutenfranz 1975	Inland		10–15	Above rest value; less experienced subject
Klimmer 1978	Navigation		30–40	Above normal values: difficult manoeuvre
	Operating/control			
Rohmert et al. 1973b	Air traffic control	120		Approach control, rush hour
Hartemann, Manigault, and Tarriere 1970	Rolling mill oper.		10–20	From begin to end of shift time
Woitowitz, Schäcke, and Woitwitz 1971	Surgeon	120	30	During operation; above routine activities
Bassan 1966	Musician/conductor	up to 150		Max. value recurring during the course of concert
Seliger, Glückmann, and Havlickova			30	Above rest value; high fluctuations
Schmale and Schmidtke 1965			50	Max. value during solo part
Haider and Groll-Knapp 1971				
Pastukhina and Vikhrieva 1968	Examination	mean 107		Over the whole period (1·5 h)
Jansen and Schubert 1973		max. 132		During problem setting
Thomas and Ellis 1972		110–140	40 per cent	Oral examination: during lecture period
			7 per cent	Above mean baseline: master's degree; Semester final examination

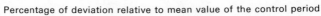

Percentage of deviation relative to mean value of the control period

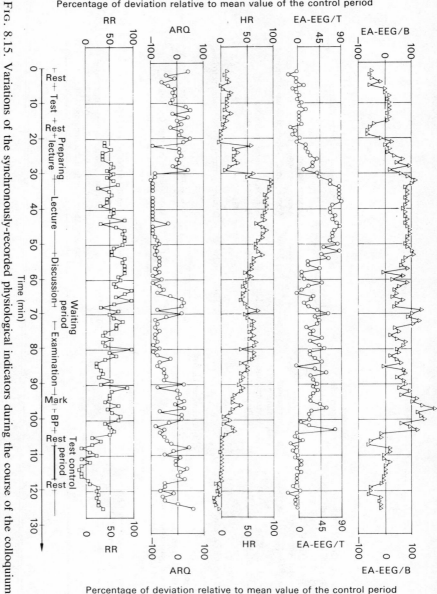

FIG. 8.15. Variations of the synchronously-recorded physiological indicators during the course of the colloquium (trial no. 4): RR = respiration rate; ARQ = scored heart-rate variability; HR = heart-rate; EA-EEG/T = EEG-theta-activity; EA-EEG/B = EEG-beta-activity.

Percentage of deviation relative to mean value of the control period

The time-dependent behaviour of the central nervous indicators shows a reaction to stressor activity with respect to the content of the task. With the beginning of the lecture theta-activity increases rapidly, followed by a steady state on a lower level until the end of the lecture. After this theta-activity decreases to a level which is maintained approximately until the end of the task. This shape of the curve with its typical reactions for emotional strain at the beginning of the task corresponds to the behaviour of heart-rate. Beta-activity shows the same rapid increase at the beginning of the lecture. The further behaviour is influenced to a greater extent by the task demand for continuous information-processing. This can be clearly seen in a higher level and lower variability during the mental arithmetic test in comparison to the neighbouring rest phases.

The behaviour of the ARQ, however, is less uniform. Whereas the decrease of the ARQ in the trial shown in Fig. 8.15 corresponds to a remarkable increase of heart-rate, in the other trials with a comparably smaller increase of heart-rate the ARQ shows a decrease, too, but only down to the level of the control period.

In Table 8.5 the results of the analysis of catecholamines for adrenalin are shown. The results show, that the adrenalin values are already increased in the period preceding the colloquium (see p. 158) (1) in comparison with the control values. This is caused by the emotional stressor component with respect to the expected stress condition. A further increase can be seen during the period of the colloquium (2), whereas the values recorded immediately following the colloquium (3) again decrease to the level of the control values.

All values recorded during the colloquium are uniformly significantly

TABLE 8.5
Urinary excretion of adrenalin ($ng\,ml^{-1}$)

Trial	n	Control measurements		Measurements under stress[1]		
		Mean values	±SD	2 h before	During	2 h after
1	8	9·90	2·57	6·3	25·8*	3·1
2	7	12·72	5·34	26·4	46·1*	10·9
3	7	10·64	6·29	23·2	46·6*	14·0
4	5	18·81	5·69	28·3	48·2*	11·9
5	7	10·97	1·25	18·6*	25·4*	14·6

[1] Taking the colloquium.
* Significant at $p = 0.05$.
Mean values and standard deviation (SD) calculated over n days during the control period.

increased in comparison to the control values (Dixon test, cited by Sachs 1968). A rank correlation between the adrenalin values for the duration of the colloquium and the recorded time series of physiological data was calculated. In the case of the physiological data, a summarizing value of the mean percentage deviation from the control period was also calculated. With a one-tailed test and a level of significance of $p = 0.05$ there is a significant positive correlation ($r_s = 0.85$) between the amount of adrenalin excretion and mean increase of heart-rate. Thus we can conclude that the increase of heart-rate under high emotional stress conditions is primarily caused by the humoral control system over adrenalin excretion. Both physiological and biochemical variables can be seen as operationally defined indicators of tonic arousal.

ARQ and respiration rate, however, do not show any significant correlation with adrenalin secretion ($r_s = -0.15$ and $r_s = 0.45$). According to the hierarchical concept of arousal a positive correlation between EEG-theta-activity and adrenalin excretion should be expected; it is, however, statistically insignificant ($r_s = 0.60$).

To elucidate the interaction between the synchronously recorded physiological indicators by means of correlation analysis the following aspects have to be taken into account. The functional unity of the organismic reactions of man according to the above-mentioned concept of arousal means that the single variables cannot be seen as independent. On the other hand interest is centred on a selective differentiation between central nervous influences and peripheral interaction mechanisms especially with respect to the 'modulation' of heart-rate and heart-rate variability (ARQ). This research interest leads to the application of partial correlation analysis to the data set. In this analysis shift time was included because in ergonomic terms it must be seen as a stress component in itself.

The results of these calculations are presented in Table 8.6, separately for the five individual cases studied. The results show that, after the elimination of intercorrelations with other variables, a positive and generally significant correlation between EEG-theta-activity and heart-rate remains; a similar positive relation to respiration rate and ARQ can be hypothesized, but cannot be statistically proven. The assessed pure correlation between EEG-beta-activity and the parameters of the cardio-respiratory system is low by comparison, but the ARQ alone shows a predominantly positive and significant correlation to EEG-beta.

The interactions between the parameters of cardio-respiratory system are characterized by predominantly negative correlations between ARQ

TABLE 8.6

Matrix of partial correlation coefficients (for abbreviations of variables, refer to text)

ARQ	HR	RR	EA-EEG/T	EA-EEG/B	
−0·17	−0·12	−0·12	0·55(s)	0·28(s)	Time
−0·14	−0·50(s)	0·14	−0·08	0·24(s)	
0·21	0·16	−0·26(s)	0·08	0·31(s)	
−0·26(s)	−0·57(s)	−0·02	0·12	0·15	
0·29(s)	−0·31(s)	0·00	−0·12	−0·13	
	0·27(s)	0·01	0·14	−0·09	ARQ
	−0·44(s)	−0·02	0·32(s)	−0·05	
	−0·08	−0·06	0·21	0·31(s)	
	−0·52(s)	−0·22(s)	0·15	0·29(s)	
	−0·24(s)	−0·23(s)	0·06	0·27(s)	
		0·02	0·19	0·11	HR
0·11	0·58(s)	0·11	0·58(s)	0·06	
		−0·03	0·42(s)	0·18	
		0·03	0·44(s)	0·04	
		0·00	0·23(s)	0·37(s)	
			−0·13	−0·03	RR
			0·09	0·03	
			0·19	0·15	
			0·02	0·25(s)	
			0·28(s)	0·04	
				−0·06	EA-EEG/T
				0·17	
				−0·16	
				0·29(s)	
				0·21(s)	

Order of trials: No. 1, 2, 3, 4, 5.
(s) level of significance: $p = 0.05$ two-tailed.

and heart-rate as well as ARQ and respiration rate, which, however, are significant in some cases only; a correlation between heart-rate and respiration rate cannot be deduced from the analyzed data. The tendencies in the relations between shift time and the other variables are heterogeneous. Only EEG-beta-activity shows a predominantly positive and significant correlation to shift time. A consequence of the positive significant correlation between EEG-theta-activity and heart-rate is a reinforcement of the thesis, that increase of heart-rate is an effect of tonic arousal.

To determine the variance in the time series of heart-rate and heart-rate variability as a function of psychophysical load, the other, synchronously recorded physiological measurements can be used as indicators according to the hierarchical concept of arousal and in accordance with the results of the correlation analysis. Thus an approach for a functional relationship has the following form:

$$\text{ARQ} = f(\text{EEG-theta, EEG-beta, HR, RR, Time})$$
$$\text{HR} = f(\text{EEG-theta, EEG-beta, Time}).$$

This approach was realized by a multiple linear regression analysis. In this analysis the error variance is minimized by a stepwise involvement of 'independent' variables, which, according to the hierarchial concept of arousal, affect the behaviour of heart-rate and heart-rate variability. The results of this stepwise multiple regression are shown in Table 8.7.

According to the results presented, the other variables can explain at minimum 20 per cent and on average 34 per cent of the time behaviour of heart-rate variability under high psychophysical load. In the hierarchical concept shift time contributes negligibly to the coefficient of determination; central nervous and peripheral physiological indicators already explain 32 per cent of variance. One-half of this component of variance, explained by physiological variables, is determined, using the hierarchical concept, by the EEG measurements, which indicate central nervous activity. The additional variance explained by EEG-beta-activity, which can be seen as reaction to the mental-informatory component of stress, is minor in comparison to the variance explained by EEG-theta-activity. This means, that under high psychophysical load, tonic arousal also has a dominant effect on heart-rate variability. In three of the five cases

TABLE 8.7

Explained variance of the time series of heart-rate (HR) and heart-rate variability (ARQ) by coefficient of determination (per cent) calculated as the square of the multiple coefficient of correlation

Trial	ARQ					HR			
	Time	HR	RR	EA-EEG/B	EA-EEG/T	EA-EEG/T	EA-EEG/B	Time	
1	47·6	45·4	18·2	15·1	12·4	22·9	39·1	55·3	
2	21·1	20·4	3·5	3·5	0·1	56·0	56·4	65·9	
3	20·2	19·6	17·3	14·7	14·3	81·0	82·7	84·7	
4	58·4	52·9	39·7	28·3	27·1	67·9	67·9	70·6	
5	20·7	19·1	18·9	17·9	16·9	37·0	44·9	45·5	
Mean	33·6	31·5	19·5	15·9	14·2	51·0	58·2	64·4	

studied, EEG-beta-activity as an indicator of phasic arousal has a negative coefficient of regression in the multiple equation. This supports the hypothesis, that a decrease of heart-rate variability under mental work load will occur. Discussing the peripheral physiological interactions, a dominant contribution to the determination of variance of ARQ is delivered by heart-rate, whereas respiration rate shows only little effect.

Within this context of the hierarchical model of arousal and stepwise multiple regression, variance of heart-rate can be explained to a greater extent by the measurements of central nervous activity, whereby more than 50 per cent of variance is determined by EEG-theta-activity. A comparison with the mean values of heart-rate calculated over the total period of the experiment, shows a tendency in the interaction between the absolute amount of heart-rate and the contribution to the coefficient of determination by EEG measurements: the component of the variance of heart-rate, which can be explained by EEG-theta, increases with the level of heart-rate itself—an effect, which can be assigned to tonic arousal. The additional component of variance, explained by EEG-beta, decreases simultaneously—that is a reduced effect of phasic arousal. In contrast, the variance of heart-rate variability, as determined by central nervous indicators of arousal, has a higher contribution to the total amount of explained variance, the lower the level of heart-rate itself is.

Discussion

With the polygraphic measurement concept a relatively high part of the variance in the reaction of the cardio-respiratory system to stress can be explained and assigned to indicators within a hierarchical arousal concept. The part of variance explained with respect to heart-rate variability is much higher than that which can be explained by the concept of superimposition of different stressors in the laboratory experiment (see §8.4, Experiment 1). On the other hand, the investigations reported show that the close relation between a decrease of heart-rate variability and external stressors—in the concept related to phasic and tonic arousal—cannot be reproduced in a field situation with high components of emotional load. Besides this emotional load the effects of speaking and body movements can be taken as reasons why heart-rate variability does not decrease to the expected extent in the reported cases. In addition to these effects, the emotional stress situation and the respective amount of tonic arousal may lead the humoral control system with increased adrenalin excretion to an '*increased* heart-rate baroreceptor reflex sensitivity' (see

167

Hyndman and Gregory 1975) as well as producing increased amplification factors in other parts of the heart-rate control system, which would mean increased oscillation with constant excitation–signal flow.

It can be supposed, that the effects of phasic arousal by neural pathways are not able to compensate this humoral effect on the heart-rate control system. In contrast to the laboratory experiment with a constant and continuous signal input and output flow with respect to the task and the constant level of phasic arousal which can be deduced from this, we assume for the field experiment, that the level of phasic arousal in the situation of an university examination varies to a greater extent as the demands of the task vary; for example, the type of questions of the professor and the audience or their reactions to answers of the candidate may vary. Thus a greater variability of phasic arousal itself may cause a greater variability in the behaviour of the recorded physiological time series.

8.6. Conclusion

From the experimental and model results as well as their confirmations in the literature the following conclusions can be drawn:

HRV decreases under mental load as is also shown by many other authors, but it is affected by endogeneous physiological functions to a greater extent than by mental load.

HRV must be carefully used as a physiological indicator of mental load if the task requires that the subjects often speak, because the pattern of respiration under speaking conditions suppresses and disturbs the mental strain reaction in HRV.

HRV should not be used as a physiological indicator of mental strain, if the motor actions for information-handling activities involve big groups of muscles. The receptors for metabolic functions within the muscles are directly coupled with heart-rate, so that even the pedalling rate when answering a binary choice task could be detected as a peak in the power spectrum of HRV.

HRV cannot be used as a measure of mental strain if heart-rate increases significantly owing to additional physical workload, metabolic, or thermal effects.

The contribution of HRV to the information about non-physical strain should be verified by a partial correlation analysis, to see if heart-rate increased significantly owing to emotional effects.

The individual reaction of each subject should be corrected by a 'range correction' proposed above in order to get interindividually comparable results. For this purpose a standardized task with non-physical load should be used to calibrate the intraindividual dynamics of HRV of the subjects, before using it as a measurement for the evaluation of field situations.

For the application of HRV in ergonomic field studies with high mental and emotional components of stress one has to take into account, that, due to the resulting high amount of tonic arousal, heart-rate variability is destroyed by 'noise'. Only if the task leads to phasic arousal and a comparably low amount of tonic arousal, can the use of heart-rate variability be suggested as a selective indicator with respect to the evaluation of strain.

In continuous recordings of instantaneous heart-rate the transistory phases between two different steps of load cannot be used for the calculation of heart-rate variability, because physiological mechanisms other than those effecting a decrease of HRV under mental load, determine momentary heart-rate.

In conclusion it can be said, that HRV is a quite good indicator of non-physical strain in the laboratory with steady state and *ceteris paribus* conditions, but it is very difficult to handle and has restricted value for the evaluation of strain in practical situations with their usually varying situational and mental load conditions.

References

ADEY, W. R. (1969). Spectral analysis of EEG data from animals and man during alerting, orienting and discriminative responses. In *Attention in neurophysiology* (eds C. R. Evans and T. B. Mulholland). Butterworth, London.

ANGELONE, A. and COULTER, N. (1964). Respiratory sinus arrhythmia: a frequency dependent phenomenon. *J. appl. Physiol.* **19**, 479–82.

ARNOLD, W. (1961). *Der Pauli-Test.* Barth, Munich.

ATTNEAVE, F. (1968). *Informationstheorie in der Psychologie.* Huber, Berne.

BALKE, B., MELTON, C. E., and BLAKE, C. (1966). Physiological stress and fatigue in aerial missions for the control of forest fires. *Aerospace Med.* **37**, 221–27.

BARTENWERFER, H. (1960). Herzrhythmik—Merkmale als Indikatoren psychischer Anspannung. *Psycholog. Beiträge* **4**, 7–25.

BASSAN, L. (1966). Über die Aussagekraft der Herzschlagfrequenz als physiologische Meßgröße in der Leistungsphysiologie. *Int. Arch. Gewerbepath. Gewerbehyg.* **22**, 262–81.

BAUMGARTEN, R. V., BALTHASAR, K., and KOEPCHEN, H. P. (1960). Über ein

Substrat atmungsrhythmischer Erregungsbildung im Rautenhirn der Katze. *Pflüger's Arch. ges. Physiol.* **270**, 504–28.

BECHTEREVA, N. P., KAMBAROVA, A. K., and POZDEEV, V. K. (1975). Emotional interrelationships of principal catecholaminergic centres in the brain. In *Catecholamines and behavior*, Vol. 1 *Basic neurobiology* (ed. A. J. Friedhoff) pp. 109–64. Plenum, London.

BENTE, D., FRICK, K., LEWINSKY, M., PENNING, J., and SCHEULER, W. (1976). Signalanalytische Untersuchungen zur Wirkung des Antidepressivums Nomifensin auf das EEG gesunder Probanden. *Arzneimit. Forsch.* **26**, 1120–5.

BLITZ, P. S., HOOGSTRATEN, J., and MULDER, G. (1970). Mental load, heart rate and heart rate variability. *Psycholog. Forsch.* **33**, 277–88.

BOYCE, P. R. (1974). Sinus arrhythmia as a measure of mental load. *Ergonomics* **17**, 177–83.

BRODAN, V., HAJEK, M., and KUHN, E. (1971). An analog model of pulse rate during physical load and recovery. *Physiol. Bohemoslovaca* **10**, 189–98.

BROICHER, H. A. and DUPUIS, H. (1963). Messverfahren für automatischen Pulsfrequenzschrieb und Anwendungsbereiche. *Int. Z. angew. Physiol.* **20**, 75–89.

CASPERS, H. (1973). Zentralnervensystem. In *Kurzgefaßtes Lehrbuch der Physiologie* (Ed. W. D. Keidel). Thieme, Stuttgart.

CLYNES, M. (1960a). Respiratory sinus arrhythmia: laws derived from computer simulation. *J. appl. Physiol.* **15**, 863–74.

—— (1960b). Respiratory heart rate control. Some non-linear control techniques, novel to control engineers, employed by a biological control system. *Proceedings of IFAC Congress, Moscow*, Vol. 2, pp. 664–73.

—— (1960c). Computer analysis of reflex control and organisation: respiratory sinus arrhythmia. *Science* **131**, 300–2.

COLES, M. G. H. (1972). Cardiac and respiratory activity during visual search. *J. exp. Psychol.* **96**, 371–9.

DANEV, S. G. and WARTNA, G. F. (1970). Information load and time stress. Some psychophysiological consequences. *TNO-Nieuws* **25**, 389–95.

—— —— and RADDER, J. J. (1971). Are the RR intervals in the ECG normally distributed? *Pflüger's Arch. ges. Physiol.* **328**, 261.

—— —— BINK, B., RADDER, J. J. and LUTEYN, I. (1972). Psychophysiological assessment of information load. *Nederland. Tijdschr. Psychol.* **26**, 23–39.

DUFFY, E. (1957). The psychological significance of the concept of 'arousal' or 'activation'. *Psychol. Rev.* **64**, 265–75.

EICHLER, J. and LOBSIEN, I. (1970). Telemetrie des Belastungs-EKG beim Sportflug. In *Biotelemetrie* (eds L. Demling and K. Bachmann). Thieme, Stuttgart.

ENGEL, P., HILDEBRANDT, G. and VOGT, E. D. (1969). Der Tagesgang der Phasenkoppelung zwischen Herzschlag und Atmung in Ruhe und seine Beeinflussung durch dosierte Arbeitsbelastung. *Int. Z. angew. Physiol.* **27**, 339–55.

ETTEMA, J. H. (1967). *Arbeidsfysiologische Aspecten van Mentale Belasting.* Van Gorcum & Co., Assen.

—— and ZIELHUIS, R. L. (1971). Physiological parameters of mental load. *Ergonomics* **14**, 137–44.

EULER VON, U. S. (1964). Ausscheidungsmuster von Katecholaminen während verschiedener physiologischer und pathophysiologischer Zustände. In *Funktionsabläufe unter emotionellen Belastungen* (ed. K. Fellinger). Karger, Basle.

FELDMAN, J. L. and COWAN, J. D. (1975a). Large-scale activity in neural nets. I. *Biol. Cybernet.* **17**, 29–38.

—— —— (1975b). Large-scale activity in neural nets. II. *Biol. Cybernet.* **17**, 39–51.

FIRTH, P. A. (1973). Psychological factors influencing the relationship between cardiac arrhythmia and mental load. *Ergonomics* **16**(1), 5–16.

FRANKENHÄUSER, M. (1969). Biochemische Indikatoren der Aktiviertheit: Die Ausscheidung von Katecholaminen. In *Methoden der Aktivierungsforschung, Psychologisches Kolloquium, VI* (ed. W. Schönpflug). Huber, Berne.

—— (1975). Experimental approaches to the study of catecholamines and emotion. In *Emotions—their parameters and measurement* (ed. L. Levi). Raven Press, New York.

FRIEDHOFF, A. J. (1975). Integration and conclusion. In *Catecholamines and Behaviour, Vol. 2, Neuropsychopharmacology* (ed. A. J. Friedhoff). Plenum, London.

GAILLARD, A. W. K. and TRUMBO, D. A. (1976). Drug effects on heart rate and heart rate variability during a prolonged reaction task. *Ergonomics* **19**(5), 611–22.

GLASER, G. H. (1963). The normal electroencephalogram and its reactivity. In *EEG and Behaviour* (ed. G. H. Glaser). Basic Books, New York.

GOLENHOFEN, K. and HILDEBRANDT, G. (1958). Die Beziehung des Blutdruckrhythmus zu Atmung und peripherer Durchblutung. *Pflüger's Arch. ges. Physiol.* **267**, 27–45.

—— —— (1961). Zur relativen Koordination von Atmung und Blutdruckwellen 3. Ordnung. *Z. Biol.* **112**, 451–8.

GRIMBY, G., NILSON, J., and SALTIN, B. (1966). Cardiac output during submaximal and maximal exercise in active middle-aged athletes. *J. appl. Physiol.* **21**, 1150–6.

HAIDER, M. (1969). Elektrophysiologische Indikatoren der Aktiviertheit. In *Methoden der Aktivierungsforschung (Psycholog. Kolloq., VI)* (ed. W. Schönpflug). Huber, Berne.

—— and GROLL-KNAPP, E. (1971). Psychophysiologische Untersuchungen über die Belastung des Musikers in einem Symphonieorchester. In *Stress und Kunst* (ed. M. Piperek). W. Braumüller, Universitäts-Verlagsbuchhandlg, Wien-Stuttgart.

HALE, H. B., WILLIAMS, E. W., and BUCKLEY, C. J. (1969). Aeromedical aspects of the first nonstop transatlantic helicopter flight: III. Endocrinemetabolic effects. *Aerospace Med.* **40**, 718–23.

HARTEMANN, F., MANIGAULT, P., and TARRIERE, C. (1970). An endeavour to evaluate the nervous load at work stations in line production. *Int. J. Production Res.* **8**(1), 3–10.

HARTUNG, M. (1966). Über die Atmungsregulation unter Arbeit. *Forschungsbericht des Landes Nordrhein-Westfalen, No.* 1738. Westdeutscher Verlag, Cologne/Opladen.

HILDEBRANDT, G. (1967). Die Koordination rhythmischer Funktionen beim Menschen. In *Verhandlungen der Deutschen Gesellschaft für innere Medizin*, 73. *Kongress* 1967. Bergmann, Munich.

HOAGLAND, H., BERGEN, J. R., BLOCH, E., ELMADJIAN, F., and GIBREE, N. R. (1955). Adrenal stress responses in normal men. *J. appl. Physiol.* **8**, 149–54.

HOFFMANN, H., STRUBEL, H., RAABE, H., and KOCH, M. (1969). Biotelemetrische Untersuchungen des Herz–Kreislauf-Systems bei Hubschrauber-Piloten zur Feststellung der unterschiedlichen fliegerischen Belastung. *Zbl. Verkehrsmed.* **15**, 1–26.

HOLMGREN, A. (1956). Arterial blood pressure during muscular work. *Scand. J. clin. lab. Invest.* **8**, 29–89.

HOLLMANN, W. (1959). *Der Arbeits- und Trainingseinfluss auf Kreislauf und Atmung.* Steinkopff, Darmstadt.

—— (1963). Höchst- und Dauerleistungsfähigkeit des Sportlers. Barth, Munich.

HORGAN, J. D. and LANGE, D. L. (1962). Analog computer studies of periodic breathing. *IRE Trans. bio-med. Electron.* **9**, 221–8.

—— —— (1964). The human respiratory system. *Simulation* **3**, 44–51.

HOWITT, J. S., BALKWILL, J. S., WHITESIDE, T. C. D., and WHITTINGSHAM, P. D. G. V. (1965). *A preliminary study of flight deck work loads in civil air transport aircraft.* Flying Personnel Research Committee, FPRC 1240, Ministry of Aviation and the Royal Air Force, Institute of Aviation Medicine, Farnborough. Ministry of Defence, Air Force Department.

HYNDMAN, B. W., KITNEY, R. J., and SAYERS, B. McA. (1971). Spontaneous rhythms in physiological control systems. *Nature* **233**, 339–41.

—— and GREGORY, J. R. (1975). Spectral analysis of sinus arrhythmia during mental loading. *Ergonomics* **18** (3), 255–70.

JANSEN, G. and SCHUBERT, A. (1973). Physiologische Messwerte und moderierende Einflussgrössen bei der ärztlichen Prüfung. In *Problematik von Arbeitsplätzen mit mentaler Belastung* (ed. H. G. Wenzel and F. J. Tentrup). 12th Annual Meeting of the Deutsche Gesellschaft für Arbeitsmedizin, 25–28 October 1972, Dortmund. Gentner, Stuttgart.

KALSBEEK, J. H. W. (1963). *Perceptieve Last en Belastbaarheid. Stuurgroep Ergonomie.* Jaarverslag, Amsterdam.

—— (1967). *Mentale Belasting.* Van Gorcum & Co., Assen.

KEIDEL, W. D. (Ed.) (1973). *Kurzgefasstes Lehrbuch der Physiologie.* Thieme, Stuttgart.

KICZKA, K. and CZYZEWSKA, E. (1976). Untersuchungen der Einmannbesatzung von Diesel-Lokomotiven. *Arbeitsmed., Sozialmed., Präv.-Med.* **11**, 292–5.

KLIMMER, F. (1978). Analyse mentaler und emotionaler Beanspruchung des arbeitenden Menschen. Dissertationschrift TH Darmstadt, Darmstadt.

KLINGER, K.-P. and STRASSER, H. (1972). Variations of physiological parameters during defined mental load and rest. *Pflüger's Arch. ges. Physiol.* **332**, R28.

KOEPCHEN, H. P. (1962a). Homöostase und Rhythmus in der Kreislauf-regulation. *Bad Oeynhauser Gespräche 5.* Springer Verlag, Berlin.

—— (1962b). *Die Blutdruckrhythmik.* Steinkopff, Darmstadt.

—— (1972). Atmungsregulation. In *Atmung* (ed. J. Piiper). Urban & Schwarzenberg, Munich.

—— and BAUMGARTEN, R. V. (1960). Entladungsmuster und vagale Beeinflussung expiratorischer Neurone im Hirnstamm der Katze. *Pflüger's Arch. ges. Physiol.* **268**, 64.

KÖTZ, H. (1968). Über Pulsfrequenzsteigerungen bei Hubschrauberpiloten als Maß für ihre Beanspruchung. *Zbl. Verkehrs-Med.* **14**, 65–70.

LAURIG, W. and PHILIPP, U. (1970). Veränderungen der Pulsfrequenzarrhythmie in Abhängigkeit von der Arbeitsschwere. *Arbeitsmed. Sozialmed. Arbeitshyg.* **5**, 184–8.

—— LUCZAK, H. and PHILIPP, U. (1971). Ermittlung der Pulsfrequenzarrhythmie bei körperlicher Arbeit. *Int. Z. angew. Physiol.* **30**, 40–51.

LEGEWIE, H., SIMONOVA, O., and CREUTZFELD, D. (1970). Telemetrische EEG-Untersuchungen in Leistungssituationen. In *Biotelemetrie* (eds L. Demling and K. Bachmann). Thieme, Stuttgart.

LEVI, L. (1972). Sympathoadrenalinmedullary responses to 'pleasant' and 'unpleasant' psychosocial stimuli. In Stress and distress in response to psychosocial stimuli (ed. L. Levi). *Acta Med. scand.* (suppl. 528) 55–73.

LEVISON, H., BARNETT, G. O., and JACKSON, W. D. (1966). Nonlinear analysis of the baroreceptor reflex. *Circulation Res.* **18**, 673–82.

LINDSLEY, D. B. (1960). Attention, consciousness, sleep and wakefulness. In *Handbook of Physiology, Section 1, Neurophysiology, III* (eds J. Field, H. W. Magoun, and V. E. Hall). American Physiology Society, Washington, D.C.

—— (1961). The reticular activating system and perceptual integration. In *Electrical stimulation of the brain* (ed. O. E. Sheer). Texas University Press, Austin.

LIPPOLD, O. C. J. (1952). The relation between integrated action potentials in human muscle and isometric tension. *J. Physiol.* **117**, 492–9.

LUCZAK, H. and LAURIG, W. (1973). An analysis of heart rate variability. *Ergonomics* **16**(1), 85–98.

—— and RASCHKE, F. (1975). Regelungstheoretisches Kreislaufmodell zur Interpretation arbeitsphysiologischer und rhythmologischer Einflüsse auf die Momentanherzfrequenz: Arrhythmie. *Biol. Cybernet.* **18**, 1–13.

LYKKEN, D. T. (1972). Range correction applied to heart rate and to GSR data. *Psychophysiol.* **9**, 373–9.

Lynn, R. (1966). Attention, arousal and the orientation reaction. Pergamon, Oxford.

Malmö, R. B. and Shagass, C. (1949). The variability of heart rate in relation to age, sex and stress. *J. appl. Psychol.* **2**, 181–4.

Mandler, G. (1967). The conditions for emotional behaviour. In *Neurophysiology and emotion* (ed. D. C. Glass). Rockefeller University Press, New York.

Mason, J. W. (1971). A re-evaluation of the concept of 'non-specifity' in stress theory. *J. psychiat. Res.* **8**, 323–33.

Miyawaki, K., Takahashi, T., and Takemura, H. (1966). *Analysis and simulation of the periodic heart rate fluctuation.* Technical report, no. 16, pp. 315–25. Osaka University.

Monod, H. (1967). La validité des mesures de fréquence cardiaque en ergonomie. *Ergonomics* **10**(5), 485–537.

Mulder, G. and Mulder-Hajonides van der Meulen, W. (1973). Mental load and the measurement of heart rate variability. *Ergonomics* **16**(1), 69–84.

Mundy-Castle, A. C. (1957). The Electroencephalogram and mental activity. *EEG clin. Neurophysiol.* **9**, 643–55.

Nicholson, A. N., Hill, L. E., Borland, R. G., and Ferres, H. M. (1970). Activity of the nervous system during the let-down, approach and landing: a study of short duration high workload. *Aerospace Med.* **41**, 436–46.

Opmeer, C. H. J. M. (1973). The information content of successive RR-interval times in the ECG. Preliminary results using factor analysis and frequency analysis. *Ergonomics* **16**(1), 105–12.

Pasmooy, C. K. (1972). Unpublished diploma thesis concerning the description of sinus arrhythmia. Report of the Laboratorium voor Ergonomische Psychologie, TNO, Amsterdam.

Pastukhina, R. I. and Vikhrieva, M. P. (1968). Changes in the cardiac activity after high emotional stress. (according to dynamic radiotelemetry). [In Russian] *Bull. eksp. biol. Med.* **66**, 14–16.

Pekkarinen, A., Castren, O., Iisalo, E., Koivusalo, M., Laihinen, A., Simola, P. E., and Thomasson, B. (1961). The emotional effect of matriculation examinations on the excretion of adrenaline, noradrenaline, 17-hydroxycorticosteroids into the urine and the content of 17-hydroxycorticosteroids in the plasma. *Biochem., Pharmacol., Physiol.* 117–137.

Pickering, W. D., Nikiforuk, P. N., and Merriman, J. E. (1969). Analogue computer model of the human cardiovascular control system. *IEEE Trans. Bio-med. Engng (Inst. elect. electron. Engrs)* **BME-7**, 401–10.

Piiper, J. (Ed.) (1972). *Atmung.* Urban & Schwarzenberg, Munich.

Porges, S. W., 1972, Heart rate variability and deceleration as indices of reaction time. *J. exp. Psychol.* **92**, 103–10.

—— and Raskin, D. C. (1969). Respiratory and heart rate components of attention. *J. exp. Psychol.* **81**, 497–503.

Randall, W. C. (1977). Sympathetic control of the heart. In *Neural regulation of the heart* (ed. W. C. Randall). Oxford University Press, New York.

Rapp, R. M., Dietlein, L. F., and Nuttall, J. C. (1965). Some physiological observations and monitoring techniques associated with auto racing. *Aerospace Med.* **36,** 159.

Reid, D. H. and Doerr, J. E. (1970). Physiological studies of military parachutists via Fm/FM telemetry: the data acquisition system and heart rate response. *Aerospace Med.* **41,** 1292–7.

Renbourn, E. T. (1962). Variation over a period of a year, in resting pulse rate and oral temperature in young men. In *Biometeorology*, Vol. 1. Pergamon, Oxford.

Renemann, H., Beckhove, P., and Roskamm, H. (1968). Herzfrequenz bei Fallschirmabsprüngen. In *Stress und Fliegen sowie aktuelle Probleme der Flugmedizin.* Vorträge der 12. Flugmedizinischen Arbeitstagung in Fürstenfeldbruck.Wehrdienst und Gesundheit, 16. Wehr und Wissen Verlagsgesellschaft, Darmstadt.

Rohmert, W. (1960). *Statische Haltearbeit des Menschen.* Beuth-Vertrieb, Berlin.

—— (1962). *Untersuchungen über Muskelermüdung und Arbeitsgestaltung. Schriftenreihe 'Arbeitswissenschaft und Praxis'* Beuth-Vertrieb, Berlin.

—— (1973). *Psycho-physische Belastung und Beanspruchung von Fluglotsen.* Beuth-Vertrieb, Stuttgart, and Gentner, Frankfurt.

—— and Luczak, H. (1973). Zur ergonomischen Beurteilung informatorischer Arbeit. *Int. Z. angew. Physiol.* **31,** 209–29.

—— Laurig, W., Philipp, U., and Luczak, H. (1973). Heart rate variability and work-load measurements. *Ergonomics* **16**(1), 33–44.

—— and Rutenfranz, J. (1975). Arbeitswissenschaftliche Beurteilung der Belastung und Beanspruchung an unterschiedlichen industriellen Arbeitsplätzen. Der Bundesminister für Arbeit und Sozialordnung, Referat Öffentlichkeitsarbeit, Bonn.

Roman, J. (1965). Risk and responsibility as factors affecting heart rate in test pilots. The flight research program-II, *Aerospace Med.* **36,** 518–23.

Routtenberg, A. (1968). The two-arousal hypothesis: reticular formation and limbic system. *Psychol. Rev.* **76,** 51–80.

Rowen, B. (1961). Biomedical monitoring of the X-15 Program. Air Force Flight Test Center, Flight Test Engineering Division, Edwards Air Force Base, AFFTC-TN-61-4, California.

Rutenfranz, J., Rohmert, W., and Iskander, A. (1971). Über das Verhalten der Pulsfrequenz während des Erlernens sensumotorischer Fertigkeiten unter besonderer Berücksichtigung der Pausenwirkung. *Int. Z. angew. Physiol.* **29,** 101–18.

Sachs, L. (1968). *Statistische Auswertungsmethoden.* Springer, Berlin.

Sadowski, Z. (1976). Fahrgeschwindigkeit und Herzfrequenz bei Lokführern. *Ärztliche Dienst* **37,** 11–12.

Sayers, B., McA. (1973). Analysis of heart rate variability. *Ergonomics* **16**(1), 17–32.

SCHER, A. M. and YOUNG, A. C. (1963). Servoanalysis of carotid sinus reflex effects on peripheral resistance. *Circulation Res.* **12,** 152–62.

SCHLOHMKA, G. (1936). Untersuchungen über die physiologische Unregelmässigkeit des Herzschlags. *Z. Kreislaufforsch.* **26**(13), 473–92.

SCHMALE, H. and SCHMIDTKE, H. (1965). Psychophysische Belastung von Musikern in Kulturorchestern. B. Schott's Söhne, Mainz.

SELIGER, V., GLÜCKMANN, J., and HAVLICKOVA, L. (1972). Bewertung der mittels Pulsfrequenz im Verlaufe eines Konzertes beobacheten Belastungen von Musikern und Dirigenten eines Symphonierorchesters. *Das Orchester* **20,** 459–64.

SHANE, W. P. and SLINDE, K. E. (1968). Continuous ECG recording during free-fall parachuting. *Aerospace Med.* **39,** 597–603.

SHARPLESS, S. and JASPER, H. (1956). Habituation of the arousal reaction. *Brain* **79,** 655–80.

SIGG, E. B. (1975). The organization and functions of the central sympathetic nervous system. In *Emotions—their parameters and measurement* (ed. L. Levi). Raven Press, New York.

SMITH, H. P. R. (1967). The effects of stress in civil transport pilots. In *Reports of the 7th Conference for Aviation Psychology* (ed. F. J. Miret y Alsira). Western European Association for Aviation Psychology, Brussels.

SOKOLOW, E. N. (1963). *Perception and the conditioned reflex.* Pergamon Press, Oxford.

STEGEMANN, J. (1963). Zum Mechanismus der Pulsfrequenzeinstellung durch den Stoffwechsel IV. *Pflüger's Arch. ges. Physiol.* **276,** 511–24.

—— (1971). *Leistungsphysiologie.* Thieme, Stuttgart.

—— and GEISEN, K. (1966a). Zur regelungstheoretischen Analyse des Blutkreislaufs II. *Pflüger's Arch. ges. Physiol.* **287,** 257–64.

—— —— (1966b). Zur regelungstheoretischen Analyse des Blutkreislaufs IV. *Pflüger's Arch. ges. Physiol.* **287,** 276–85.

—— GOTKE, M., and GEISEN, K. (1966). Zur regelungstheoretischen Analyse des Blutkreislaufs III. *Pflüger's Arch. ges. Physiol.* **287,** 265–75.

—— and MÜLLER-BÜTOW, H. (1966). Zur regelungstheoretischen Analyse des Blutkreislaufs I. *Pflüger's Arch. ges. Physiol.* **287,** 247–56.

STRASSER, H. (1974). Beurteilung ergonomischer Fragestellungen mit Herzfrequenz und Sinusarrhythmie. *Int. Arch. Arbeitsmed.* **32,** 261–87.

THOMAS, R. E. and ELLIS, N. C. (1972). An analysis of the situational stresses of university students as measured by heart rate. In *Proceedings of the 16th Annual Meeting of the Human Factors Society 1972* (ed. W. D. Knowles) The Human Factors Society, Santa Monica, California.

WAGNER, R. (1954). *Probleme und Beispiele biologischer Regelung.* Thieme, Stuttgart.

WARTNA, G. F., DANEV, S. G., and BINK, B. (1971). Heart rate variability and mental load. A comparison of different scoring methods. *Pflüger's Arch. ges. Physiol.* **328,** 262.

WEIDINGER, H. and LESCHHORN, V. (1964). Sympathische Tonisierung und rhythmische Blutdruckschwankungen. *Z. Kreislaufforsch.* **53,** 925–1002.

WIERSMA, E. D. (1913). Der Einfluss von Bewusstseinszuständen auf den Puls und auf die Atmung. *Z. gesamt. Neurol. Psychiat.* **19,** 1.

WOITOWITZ, H. J., SCHÄCKE, G., and WOITOWITZ, R. (1971). Zur Erfassung psycho-vegetativer Belastungen am Arbeitsplatz mit Hilfe der Radiotelemetrie. *Arbeitsmed., Sozialmed. Arbeitshyg.* **6**(10), 259–62.

WOMACK, B. F. (1971). The analysis of respiratory sinus arrhythmia using spectral analysis and digital filtering. *IEEE Trans. Bio-med. Engng (Inst. elect. electron. Engrs)* **BME-18,** 399–409.

ZWAGA, H. J. G. (1973). Psychophysiological reaction to mental tasks: effort or stress? Ergonomics **16**(1), 61–8.

9.
Heart-rate changes in test pilots
A. H. ROSCOE

9.1. Introduction

FOR more than eight years test pilots at the Royal Aircraft Establishment, Bedford have had their heart-rates recorded while flying experimental sorties. The results, together with subjective ratings by the pilots, have been used to estimate and to compare levels of workload.

The term workload is vague and tends to be interpreted according to one's own discipline and interests so a few words of explanation may be helpful. Several authors have found it useful to consider workload as three functionally related factors based on:

  (i) Analysis of the task;
 (ii) Analysis or assessment of operator effort;
(iii) Analysis or measurement of results or performance (Jahns 1973; Billings and Lauber 1975).

These factors can conveniently be thought of as three major or primary facets of a multifaceted concept. Minor or subsidiary facets may be formed by the many different methods or techniques available for analysing primary factors.

From the point of view of experimental test flying, the second major facet, operator or pilot effort, seems to be the most appropriate. In addition, this way of interpreting workload caters for individual variations in such characteristics as natural ability, training, experience, age, and fitness. It is also the concept of workload to which most pilots would subscribe. For example, Cooper and Harper (1969) defined pilot workload as 'the integrated physical and mental effort required to perform a specified piloting task'. Jenny and his colleagues (1972) suggested that workload is 'the level of effort required to perform a given activity or complex of tasks'. In this context, it seems reasonable to assess workload by asking the pilot for his subjective opinion and to augment it by measuring his physiological activity. By referring to examples from flight and simulator trials, this chapter briefly describes the practical use of heart-rate and discusses the possible use of sinus arrhythmia in assessing workload.

9.2. Heart-rate as a measure of pilot workload

Flying a modern transport aircraft requires very little physical effort and the job has been classed as light or sedentary work by various authors (Littell and Joy 1969). However, considerable mental effort may be involved during the more demanding phases of flight such as take-off and the landing approach. The latter manoeuvre in particular, generates a high level of workload and so it is not surprising that some 40 to 50 per cent of accidents occur at this time. It would be wrong, though, to infer that high levels of workload are always implicated as there is plenty of evidence to suggest that low workload, leading to complacency, is sometimes a causative factor in accidents. Nevertheless, the introduction of new techniques and systems associated with take-off, and with approach and landing, must not generate unacceptable levels of workload.

At Bedford, a large area of research is concerned with approach and landing. Assessing levels of pilot workload is important in evaluating new flight systems and techniques associated with this phase of flight. Heart-rate is normally plotted as a beat-to-beat rate against time, along with the basic ECG signal from which it is derived. After visual inspection of the traces manual analysis is used to give mean rates for consecutive 30-s epochs (Fig. 9.1). This particular time interval was chosen because it seemed long enough to minimize the effect of sinus arrhythmia but short enough to allow us to recognize meaningful changes in heart-rate. Subsequent experience has supported the choice of this epoch length. Visual examination and manual analysis of the beat-to-beat plots, though tedious, is well worth the extra time and effort involved because of the amount of useful information available in the raw data which would tend to be lost by using computer-aided techniques.

The use of in-flight heart-rate measurement of test pilots is illustrated by referring to recent flight trials concerned with reducing noise on the landing approach. One way in which noise can be reduced is by flying the aircraft down a steeper slope. Gradients up to and including 9° have been investigated in detail, using different types of aircraft. Not surprisingly, heart-rate levels increased with increased rates of descent caused by steeper approach angles. By introducing a 3°-segment at the lower end of a steep slope a little of the noise reduction is sacrificed but heart-rates are

179

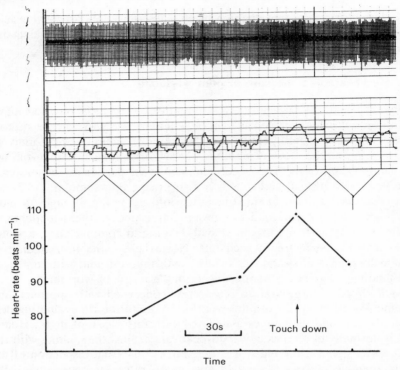

FIG. 9.1. ECG (upper trace), beat-to-beat heart-rate (middle trace), and the derived 30-s heart-rate obtained from a BAC 1-11 pilot during approach and landing.

maintained at similar levels to those for conventional 3°-approaches. The advantage of this profile can be seen in Fig. 9.2 which shows the heart-rate response for a pilot flying a BAC VC-10 airliner. Mean levels for eighteen 5°- and 6°-single-segment approaches and landings are compared with those for eleven 5°/3°-'double-flare' approaches and landings. In this particular example there was little difference between the 5°- and 6°-gradients and they have been combined.

In these double-flare approaches and landings the 3°-slope was intersected at 150 ft, but a further lowering of heart-rate occurred when the lower segment was started at 500 ft: the two-segment approach proper. Fig. 9.3 compares mean heart-rate responses for twelve 5°/3°-two-segment approaches and landings with those for six conventional 3°-approaches and landings.

180

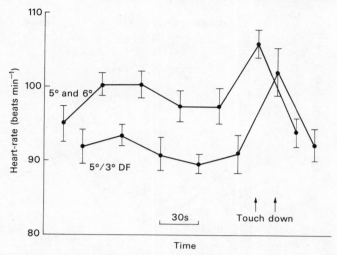

FIG. 9.2. Comparison of (30-s) mean heart-rates (±standard deviation) for 5°- and 6°-single-segment ($n = 18$), with 5°/3° 'double flare' ($n = 11$) visual approaches and landings (VC-10).

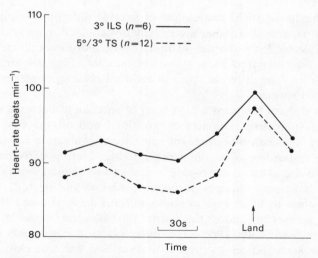

FIG. 9.3. Comparison of (30-s) mean heart-rates for 5°/3° two-segment ($n = 12$) with 3° ILS ($n = 6$) approaches and landings (VC-10).

181

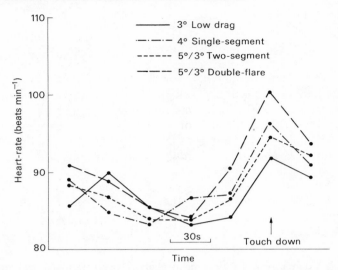

FIG. 9.4. Comparison of (30-s) mean heart-rates ($n = 4$) for four types of approaches and landings (VC-10).

After the initial flight evaluation of several different techniques and modifications, a small number are usually investigated in more detail. It is then possible to design sorties so that two or more experimental conditions can be compared in a statistical manner. Fig. 9.4 shows mean heart-rates for four different types of reduced noise approaches flown on each of four sorties.

In general there has been a high level of agreement between heart-rate values and subjective estimates of workload and on the few occasions when there has been disagreement subsequent evaluation has shown the heart-rate responses to be the more reliable. During early exploratory studies into the value of heart-rate as a measure of pilot workload it was apparent that minor changes in mental load may not be reflected by an overall change in heart-rate. Various authors have stressed the advantages of measuring more than one physiological variable (Benson, Huddleston, and Rolfe 1965). However, practical constraints precluded monitoring such indices as muscle tension and galvanic skin response; because of the frequent use of voice communication in test flying, the recording of the respiratory rate was considered to be unreliable.

9.3. Sinus arrhythmia as a measure of pilot workload

In 1968 Kalsbeek suggested the possibility of using sinus arrhythmia as a measure of pilot workload. He pointed out though, that the variability may be suppressed by an increase in over-all rate as well as by an increase in mental load and that it may be impossible to differentiate between the two effects. Sinus arrhythmia was therefore investigated as a sensitive measure of workload for use on occasions when changes in over-all heart-rate did not occur. At that time a fairly simple technique was used in which heartbeats were recorded as audio pulses and analysis was simply accomplished by counting the number of 'bleeps' in 30-s intervals. Beat-to-beat rate was obtained by using a pulse interval timer with the output, on eight-hole paper tape, being eventually processed and plotted by computer. Unfortunately, this time-consuming procedure, together with a shortage of computer time, meant that there was always a delay before beat-to-beat plots were available for inspection. Nevertheless, sinus arrhythmia seemed to hold out some promise as an indicator of mental load and, as it was available as a bonus measure, interest continued.

Fig. 9.5 is of an early beat-to-beat heart-rate plot and shows the response of a pilot during take-off in a BAC 221 supersonic research aircraft. It can be seen that heart-rate increased quite rapidly as the pilot checked essential instruments and, presumably, as his arousal level increased to prepare for the demands of the task. After starting the take-off

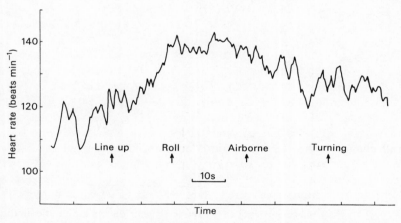

FIG. 9.5. Beat-to-beat heart-rate of a BAC 221 pilot during take-off.

run and as soon as he had correct indications of engine function and normal control response, his heart-rate fell for a few seconds before rising again at lift-off. Once airborne, there was a marked fall in heart-rate and an increase in variability. This is a typical response for a pilot taking-off in a high-performance jet aircraft.

Heart-rate responses during two automatic landings in a Comet aircraft are shown in Fig. 9.6. The upper plot is of an approach and landing with the autopilot disconnected after touchdown ready for a manual take-off. In the lower plot a poor aircraft position and attitude necessitated premature disconnection of the autopilot for a manual landing. It is quite obvious from examining these results that the marked rise in heart-rate makes the quantification of sinus arrhythmia very difficult and, from the practical point of view, unnecessary for assessing workload.

During early studies, it was usual for only one pilot at a time to be monitored but during sorties of automatic landings in poor visibility both pilot and co-pilot were monitored simultaneously. Somewhat unexpectedly, heart-rate levels remained fairly low throughout with only slight increases coinciding with marker beacons sited on the approach path. In Fig. 9.7 two pilots, flying a Vickers Varsity, alternated between captain

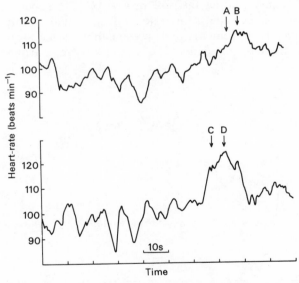

FIG. 9.6. Beat-to-beat heart-rate of a Comet 3b pilot during automatic landings: (A) land; (B) manual take-over; (C) manual take-over; (D) land.

184

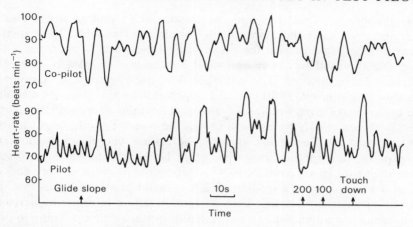

FIG. 9.7. Beat-to-beat heart-rates of a Vickers Varsity co-pilot and pilot during automatic landing in fog.

and co-pilot during twelve consecutive automatic landings in real fog. This plot and similar plots, showed periods of decreased variability without appreciable increases in overall rate.

The relative effects of different workload levels on two pilots is interesting, especially during difficult approaches and landings when the effort of the co-pilot can markedly reduce the demands on the handling pilot. Unlike the over-all heart-rate response of the latter, which invariably increases towards touchdown, the response of the co-pilot tends to remain relatively level. Yet it is known that his mental load should vary during an approach according to the demands of various operational procedures. Heart-rate plots from both pilots during autopilot approaches and from co-pilots during normal approaches provided the opportunity to evaluate sinus arrhythmia.

Using both Kalsbeek's hand scoring technique (Kalsbeek and Ettema 1963), and calculating standard deviations of interbeat heart-rate for 30-s epochs, a number of plots were analysed and levels of mental load estimated. Though the decrease in variability clearly differentiated between the different levels of mental activity according to expected changes associated with monitoring and information-processing, there was a noticeable lack of consistency.

Other workers had also failed to show a consistent relationship between load and variability when heart-rate was recorded in the field and it was decided to study evidence from a better controlled experiment using

185

several subjects. About this time, heart-rates of 75 visiting airline pilots were recorded while they were 'flying' an aircraft simulator. The experiment was designed to give the pilots some experience of approaches in poor visibility and to obtain statistical information of pilot reaction to different fog sequences. The autopilot flew the approach to a pre-set decision height of either 100 or 65 ft at which time the pilot, if he could see the runway lights, would take over and land the aircraft. If the lights were not seen clearly by decision height the co-pilot would take control for an overshoot. Each pilot, after familiarization, completed two lots of six experimental approaches during which his heart-rate was monitored. Individual runs lasted from 90 to 95 s, depending on whether they ended in an overshoot or in a landing. The command pilot's task was one of increasing vigilance followed by a decision based on information derived from visual conditions which were varied from run to run according to the experimental design. One particular visual sequence was repeated three times for each subject to detect evidence of learning. Heart-rate values were compared for two fixed periods: the first, early on the approach was used as a baseline and the second period included the decision height and the onset of the subsequent overshoot or landing.

Previous experiments with Bedford test pilots flying the simulator had resulted in minimal changes in over-all heart-rate and it was hoped therefore, that the value of sinus arrhythmia could be assessed by quantifying a large number of beat-to-beat plots obtained in carefully controlled conditions. Surprisingly, all pilots showed an over-all mean increase in heart-rate of 5 per cent or more (an example is illustrated in Fig. 9.8), though a number of individual runs did not result in any over-all change in heart-rate (Fig. 9.9). The latter results were examined and the arrhythmia scored for the two periods of each run. Visual inspection of the plots indicated when the mental load increased (revealed by a suppression of arrhythmia) but again there was a noticeable lack of consistency.

Despite being unable to quantify sinus arrhythmia in a meaningful way, heart-rate data is still displayed in a beat-to-beat format and two examples from recent flight trials are illustrated here. The first, (Fig. 9.10), is a plot of heart-rate from a pilot flying a P1127 VTOL fighter, showing a vertical take-off, an accelerating transition into normal flight, then a decelerating transition to the hover folllowed by a vertical landing. Fig. 9.11 shows plots of two pilots during an approach and landing in a BAC 1–11; changes in arrhythmia are clearly seen in spite of the much smaller amplitude available on a multiple-track recording.

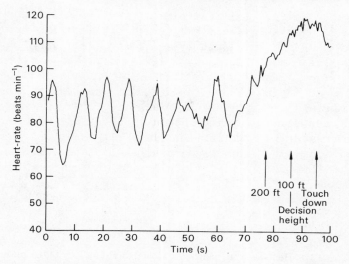

FIG. 9.8. Beat-to-beat heart-rate during simulated automatic approach, ending in a landing.

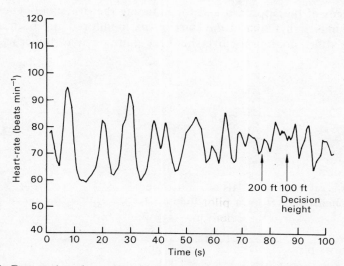

FIG. 9.9. Beat-to-beat heart-rate during simulated automatic approach, ending in an overshoot.

187

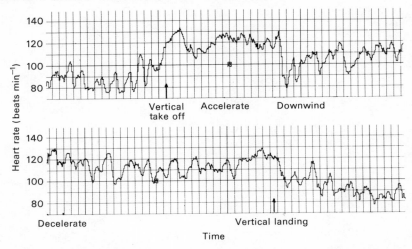

Fɪɢ. 9.10. Beat-to-beat heart-rate of a HS P-1127 (VTOL) pilot.

Occasionally a sortie consists of several similar runs and Fig. 9.12 illustrates tracings of six consecutive plots from the co-pilot during autopilot approaches in a HS 748. Each run ended in an overshoot flown by the command pilot but the co-pilot was responsible for monitoring the final stages of the approach and for initiating the overshoot. The reduction in sinus arrhythmia at the start of the monitored approach and the increase after initiating the overshoot are quite obvious. Superficially the

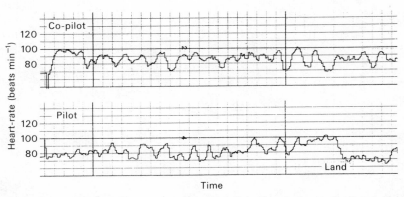

Fɪɢ. 9.11. Beat-to-beat heart-rates of a BAC 1-11 co-pilot and pilot during an approach and landing.

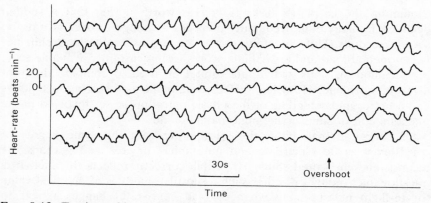

FIG. 9.12. Tracings of heart-rate of a HS 748 pilot during six consecutive runs of an automatic approach.

amount of reduction is similar for all runs, but by scoring the arrhythmia inconsistencies are revealed.

Several authors have commented adversely on the use of heart rate *per se* as the sole measure of workload. As so many factors can influence cardiovascular responses this criticism may sometimes be justified. However, most studies have been carried out in laboratories and in flight-simulators where results frequently tend to be ambiguous. On the other hand, heart-rate responses in real flight are usually meaningful and, providing that the task is well defined and realistically demanding, can often be related to levels of workload.

It is important that each pilot is used as his own control and it is desirable that during experimental runs performance be monitored and observed to be within previously defined limits. It is also advantageous to have some form of datum or standard with which to compare experimental heart-rate values. Whenever possible, it is best to compare variables within the same sortie and to fly the series according to a statistical design, such as the Latin square.

9.4. Conclusion

In practice, changes in over-all heart-rate are valuable for comparing workload levels of handling pilots during such phases of flight as the approach and landing (Roscoe 1975, 1976). Sinus arrhythmia is more sensitive and may detect changes in workload which do not result in any variation in over-all heart-rate; this may be particularly helpful in

189

evaluating the co-pilot's task. It is also worth noting that a sudden decrease in arrhythmia frequently precedes a change in over-all rate by several seconds. Unfortunately, due to an inconsistent relationship between mental load and arrhythmia scores (using currently available scoring techniques), sinus arrhythmia cannot be used to compare different levels of workload. However, further development of scoring techniques and a better understanding of the physiological processes involved in the phenomenon of sinus arrhythmia may alter this.

Of course, human pilots do not operate with the same degree of consistency as do electronic and mechanical devices and perhaps the inconsistency in scored sinus arrhythmia correctly reflects this fact. It is questionable, though, whether such a sensitive index is of practical value for in-flight measurement when over-all heart-rate changes appear to indicate realistic changes in workload.

References

BENSON, A. J., HUDDLESTON, H. F., and ROLFE, J. M. (1965). A psychophysiological study of compensatory tracking on a digital display. *Human Factors* **7** (5), 457–72.

BILLINGS, C. E. and LAUBER, J. K. (1975). Short-term workload in airline operations. *IATA Conference on 'safety in flight operations'*, Istanbul. Not published.

COOPER, G. E. and HARPER, R. P. (1969). *The use of pilot rating in the evaluation of aircraft handling qualities.* NASA Technical Note, TN.D-5153, Washington D.C.

JAHNS, D. W. (1973). *A concept of operator workload in manual vehicle operation.* Forschungsinstitut für Anthropotechnik Forschunsbericht No. 14, Meckenheim.

JENNEY, L. L., OLDER, H. J., and CAMERON, B. J. (1972). *Measurement of operator workload in an information processing task.* NASA Contractor Report CR 2150, Washington, D.C.

KALSBEEK, J. W. H. (1968). Objective measurement of mental workload: possible applications to the flight task. In *Conference proceedings No. 55: Problems of the cockpit environment.* AGARD, Paris.

—— and ETTEMA, J. H. (1963). Scored irregularity of the heart pattern and the measurement of perceptual or mental load. *Ergonomics* **6** (3), 306–7.

LITTELL, D. E. and JOY, R. J. T. (1969). Energy cost of piloting fixed and rotary-wing aircraft. *J. appl. Physiol.* **26** (3), 282–5.

ROSCOE, A. H. (1975). Heart rate monitoring of pilots during steep gradient approaches. *Aviat. Space Environ. Med.* **46** (11), 1410–3.

—— (1976). Pilot workload during steep gradient approaches. In *Conference proceedings No. 212: Aircraft operational experience and its impact on safety and survivability.* AGARD, Paris.

10.
Cardiovascular recovery to psychological stress: a means to diagnose man and task?
B. W. HYNDMAN

10.1. Introduction

THERE is ever increasing evidence that psychosocial environment is a major factor in the aetiology of essential hypertension. As Levi (1971) has pointed out, man's phylogenetically old adaptation patterns, preparing the organism for defence, have probably become inadequate, and even harmful, in response to the predominantly psychological and socio-economic stressors prevalent in modern society. The physiological intricacies of the discoordination of the defence response in these circumstances have recently been reviewed by Gilmore (1974).

In spite of the realization that a preventive emphasis in medicine demands that such factors be taken into account, there have been relatively few quantitative studies on the effect of psychological stress on cardiovascular regulatory processes in man. This may be due to the fact that invasive measurements, particularly intra-arterial blood-pressure, are precluded by the psychosomatic effects of catheterization.

Of the relatively few non-invasive cardiovascular measurements, the electrocardiogram is by far the most accessible and reliable. It is for these rather practical reasons that for the last few years we have been developing methods to extract information about the activity of cardiovascular regulatory processes from this signal (Hyndman and Mohn 1975). We have confined our studies to the R-wave spike-train of the ECG because such waves conveniently define the occurrence of a cardiac event, i.e. a heartbeat, and the timing of these events is strongly influenced by the cyclic activity of various autonomic regulatory processes via the autonomic nervous system. The classical term for this phenomenom is sinus arrhythmia.

10.2. Signal-processing of the cardiac event sequence

Fig. 10.1(a) is a model of pacemaker frequency control by autonomic nervous control of the slope of diastolic depolarization (Hyndman and

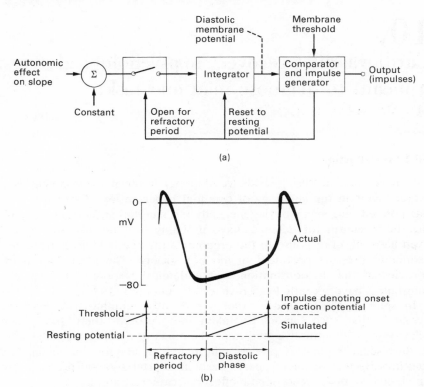

FIG. 10.1. (a) Proposed model of autonomic control of pacemaker frequency; (b) showing the aspect of actual pacemaker potential which is simulated by the model.

Mohn 1975). It has been assumed that rapid changes in autonomic activity can change the diastolic slope even within a single diastolic phase. The cell cluster constituting the pacemaker is modelled as a single effective cell, because the individual cells are electrically synchronized. The model simulates only the diastolic phase of pacemaker potential, as shown in Fig. 10.1(b), since the only aspect of action potential of interest here is its time of onset. The diastolic depolarization is simulated by integrating a constant term with one that represents the effect of autonomic activity on the diastolic slope. When this integral exceeds a fixed threshold, an impulse is generated that denotes the onset of an action potential, and the integrator is reset to the membrane resting potential potential for the refractory period.

192

When the refractory period is zero (it has been shown (Hyndman and Mohn 1975) that the presence of a finite refractory period has little influence on modulation fidelity), the behaviour of the model is identical to that of an integral pulse frequency modulator (IPFM) (Bayley 1968). Fig. 10.2 illustrates the operation of such a modulator. The input modulating signal, $X_1(t)$, and a constant term which determines the free-running or carrier frequency, are integrated with all initial conditions zero. When this integral reaches a fixed threshold value, an impulse

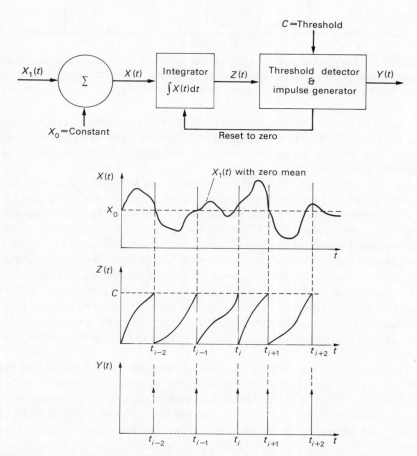

FIG. 10.2. Integral pulse frequency modulator (IPFM) which encodes a signal $X_1(t)$ into an impulse train $Y(t)$.

193

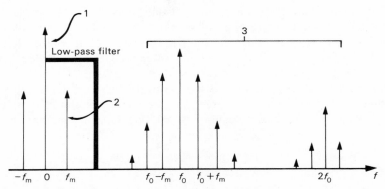

FIG. 10.3. Spectrum of output pulse train of an IPFM for a small sinusoidal input signal. If the input signal's amplitude and frequency are small enough, it can be retrieved from the output pulse train by low-pass filtering.

occurs. The larger the X-value, the sooner the threshold is reached and the impulse generated. The integrator is then reset to zero but not held there. This process is repeated, thereby encoding the input signal into an impulse train.

Fig. 10.3 shows the amplitude spectrum of an IPFM impulse train with a small sinusoidal input signal. The d.c. component, 1, is accompanied by a single component, 2, at the modulation frequency. The spectrum also contains components at all harmonics of the carrier frequency, each accompanied by an infinite set of sidebands that are removed from these harmonics by multiples of the modulation frequency. When the modulating signal's amplitude and frequency are small enough, the spread of each set of sidebands will be so limited that the imput component will be isolated. This can then be retrieved by low-pass filtering the impulse train, as shown. The cut-off frequency of the filter must be greater than the modulation frequency but lower than any sideband component of significant amplitude.

To prevent spectral biasing, the spectral window for the filtering of Fig. 10.4(a) was chosen, and the corresponding weighting function as in Fig. 10.4(b). The value of the resultant low-passed signal at a particular point in time is determined digitally by centring the weighting function at that point, and summing the weighting coefficients for previous and future impulses. To achieve a fairly rectangular spectral window, as shown in Fig. 10.4(c), it is necessary to consider only the impulses that are less than ten cycles of the weighting function distant. To avoid aliasing, the

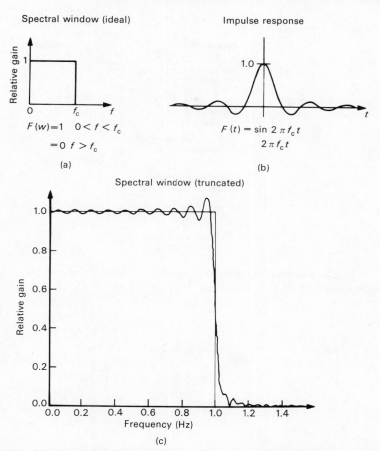

FIG. 10.4. (a) The desired frequency profile of the digital filter; (b) the corresponding weighting function (impulse response), however, exists for all time past and future; (c) the actual frequency profile when the weighting function is truncated to 20 cycles.

adjacent sample of the low-passed signal is determined by moving the centre of the weighting function at most $1/(2f_c)$ s, where f_c is the cut-off frequency of the filter, and summing the coefficients as before. This procedure produces a regularly sampled signal that can be Fourier analysed.

Actual cardiac records are processed as shown in Fig. 10.5. The R wave of the human ECG is used to define a cardiac event, the latter being

195

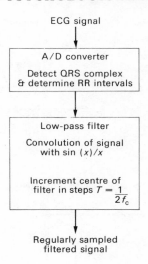

FIG. 10.5. The sequence of operations required to retrieve the information in the RR intervals of an ECG signal.

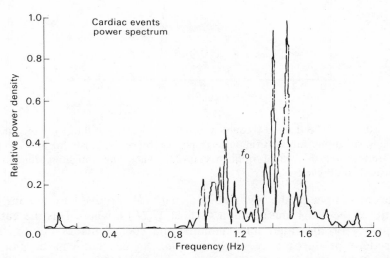

FIG. 10.6. The spectral power density of a subject's cardiac event sequence when the subject is breathing sinusoidally. The sideband components distributed about the mean heartbeat frequency, f_0, are well clear of the 'signal' component, A.

196

represented as a single impulse. A given record of events is low-pass filtered, and the regularly sampled signal is Fourier analysed.

Fig. 10.6 shows a portion of the power spectrum of a human cardiac event sequence. An approximately sinusoidal disturbance in blood-pressure, and thus in autonomic activity, produced the isolated component, A. The amplitude and frequency distribution of the cluster of components distributed about the mean heartbeat frequency, f_0, parallels

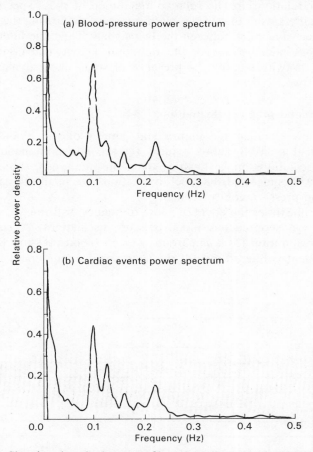

FIG. 10.7. Showing that the low-pass filtered cardiac even sequence corresponds to the autonomic signal controlling pacemaker frequency. The low-frequency spectrum of the blood-pressure (a) is very similar to that of the cardiac event sequence (b).

197

those of an IPFM with a moderate input signal. Since these components do not extend into the spectral domain of the disturbance signal, this signal can be retrieved by low-pass filtering the cardiac event sequence.

Fig. 10.7 shows the similarity of the low-frequency power spectra of the blood-pressure and cardiac event sequence in a resting, spontaneously breathing, subject. The spectral peaks in the event spectrum correspond in frequency to those in the blood-pressure spectrum, thereby indicating a fairly linear relationship.The relative magnitude of these spectral peaks somewhat differs from that of the blood-pressure, indicating the presence of some linear dynamics between the two signals. Thus, the filtered event sequence does indeed correspond to autonomic activity converging on the pacemaker, notwithstanding the presence of some linear dynamics connecting the two.

10.3. The blood-pressure fluctuations

Let us now examine the nature and genesis of the blood-pressure fluctuations. Fig. 10.8 shows typical ten-second spontaneous blood-pressure oscillations in a healthy man during apnea (breath-hold). Wagner (1950) suggested that such oscillations are feedback oscillations of the blood-pressure control system.

Fig. 10.9 illustrates the effect of a low-frequency disturbance, voluntary respiration, on spontaneous blood-pressure oscillations. A component related to respiration (b) is apparent in mean blood-pressure (c). When this component is filtered out (d) the spontaneous component remains.

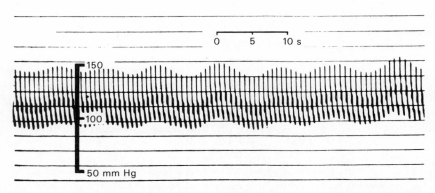

FIG. 10.8. Spontaneous 'ten-second' oscillations in human blood pressure during breath-hold.

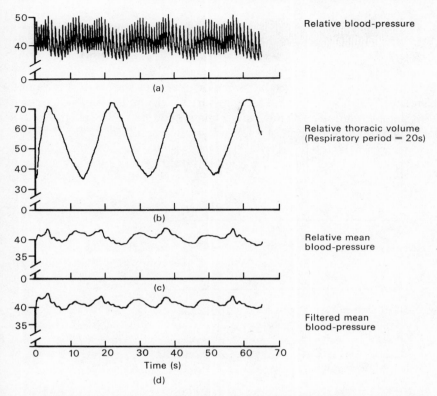

Fɪɢ. 10.9. The effect of a low-frequency disturbance (voluntary respiration) on spontaneous blood-pressure oscillation. (a) Relative blood-pressure; (b) relative thoracic volume (respiratory period = 20 s); (c) relative mean blood-pressure; (d) high-pass filtered blood-pressure, showing only the effect of the disturbance on the oscillation.

By contrast, Fig. 10.10 shows the effect of a high-frequency disturbance of the same amplitude. Only a small component related to respiration (b) is apparent in mean blood-pressure (c), and when this has been filtered out (d), no spontaneous component is evident.

The external periodic disturbance required to eliminate the spontaneous component is much larger for frequencies far below that of spontaneous oscillation than for those close to, or even much greater. This phenomenon is denoted 'frequency-selective entrainment' (FSE).

The non-linear servo-mechanism depicted in Fig. 10.11 (Hyndman

199

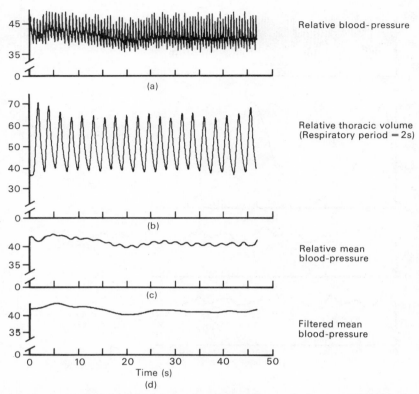

FIG. 10.10. The effect of a high-frequency disturbance (voluntary respiration) on spontaneous blood-pressure oscillation. (a) Relative blood-pressure; (b) relative thoracic volume (respiratory period = 2 s); (c) relative mean blood-pressure; (d) low-pass filtered blood-pressure showing only the effect of the disturbance on the spontaneous oscillation.

1974) can simulate two important features of the blood-pressure control system, viz., bounded spontaneous oscillations and FSE. The gain of the threshold element to the spontaneous component is inversely proportional to the disturbance for each disturbance frequency. Therefore, a sufficiently large disturbance will reduce the gain below that required, according to the Nyquist criterion, to support spontaneous oscillations. Furthermore, if, as shown in the lower panel, the frequency response of the filter circles in towards the origin with increasing frequency, the servo-mechanism displays FSE.

200

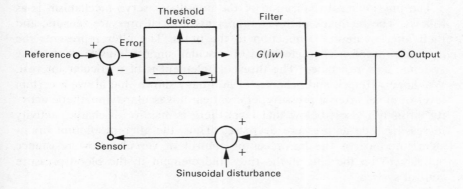

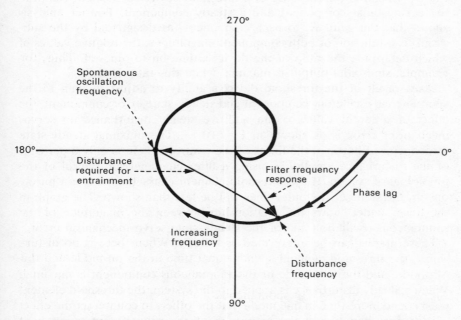

FIG. 10.11. Proposed model of blood-pressure control. The physiological realization of each element is discussed in the text. Mathematical analysis reveals how accurate regulation and spontaneous rhythms are inextricably related. 'Frequency-selective entrainment' is explained schematically below with the aid of a Nyquist plot. (See also Chapter 5.)

201

The physiological realization of the non-linear servo-mechanism is as follows. The feedback pathway represents arterial pressure sensors, and their afferent neural connection to the brain. The filter represents the dynamic response characteristics of vascular smooth muscle controlling systemic flow resistance. The threshold element is of particular interest. Weidinger, Hetzel, and Schaefer (1962) have shown that above a certain level of mean arterial pressure, efferent cardiovascular sympathetic activity virtually ceases; below that level there is massive discharge, activity increasing little as pressure decreases. Thus, the afferent/efferent brain-stem interface of the baroreceptor control of vascular flow resistance appears to be the site of the threshold element in the blood-pressure control system.

The precise homeostasis achieved by this physiological control system is also provided by the systems structure that produces the oscillations. Fig. 10.12 shows the response of a threshold device to an input comprising a sinusoidal component and a steady component. Fourier analysis shows that the gain, K, to each component (as designated by the subscript) is a function of both component magnitudes, the relative values of which determine the ratio of the device's time-on to time-off. Thus, for example, sinusoidal output is maximal when this ratio is unity.

As a result of the threshold device's ability to adjust its gain to the spontaneous oscillatory component and steady-state error component, the effect of different values of an additive steady disturbance on servo-mechanism error is as shown in Fig. 10.13. The maximal steady-state error incurred between the limits of the control system is only 6 per cent of the disturbance amplitude, using a filter characteristic typical of the physiological system. If the threshold element characteristic is not purely on–off, the slope of the outer lines will be less than shown. The graph in the lower panel shows the relationship between the magnitude of the spontaneous oscillation and of the steady-state servo-mechanism error.

These graphs can be interpreted as follows. When there is no disturbance, the threshold element spends equal time in the on-mode and the off-mode, and the amplitude of the spontaneous component is maximal. When a steady disturbance is applied to the system, the threshold element must spend more time in one mode that the other, to counteract the effect of the disturbance, and the amplitude of the spontaneous component decreases.

Thus the control systems structure responsible for the spontaneous rhythmic activity of blood-pressure also ensures the precise homeostasis of blood-pressure, and, the key element is a threshold response of

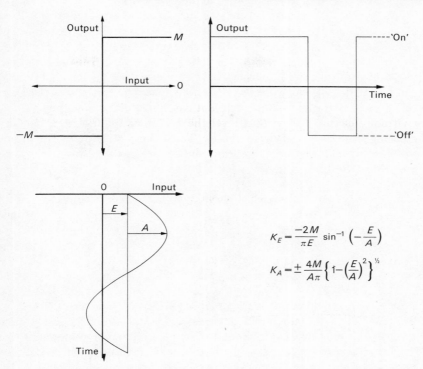

$$K_E = \frac{-2M}{\pi E} \sin^{-1}\left(-\frac{E}{A}\right)$$

$$K_A = \pm \frac{4M}{A\pi}\left\{1-\left(\frac{E}{A}\right)^2\right\}^{\frac{1}{2}}$$

Fig. 10.12. Threshold device (pure 'on–off') transfer characteristics. Fourier analysis shows that the gain of the device to a sinusoid—when both the sinusoid and a steady input are present—depends on the magnitude of both; similarly for the gain to the steady component.

efferent sympathetic nervous activity to the controlled variable, viz., mean arterial blood-pressure.

A computer simulation incorporating specific human physiological details, while retaining the over-all structural features of the general servo-mechanism model will now be examined to illustrate how the operation of such a detailed model (Hyndman 1973) parallels that of the general model. Beneken's (1965) model of the uncontrolled human cardio-vascular system, modified to include orthostasis and other factors, was used to simulate the controlled object.

Subprograms were developed to simulate baroreceptor reflexes and to control certain parameters of this hydraulic system model. The entire

203

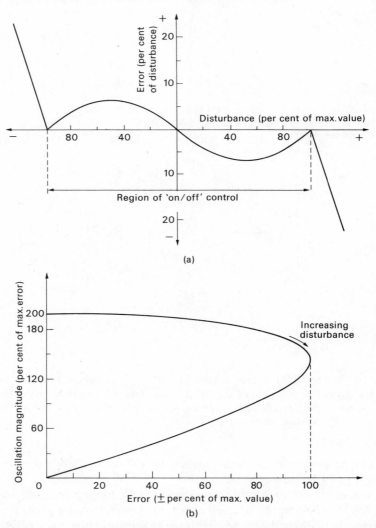

(a)

(b)

Fig. 10.13. (a) The relationship between error and disturbance for the model of Fig. 10.11. When the range of on–off control is exceeded, error increases proportionately with disturbance. If the non-linear element is not pure 'on–off', error increase will be somewhat less outside the on–off range. (b) The inextricable relationship between spontaneous rhythms and regulation accuracy.

204

model was simulated digitally. The 'cardiac interval reflex model' (Snyder and Rideout 1969), to characterize pacemaker control, was incorporated. Atrial systole is initiated when a fixed threshold is exceeded by the integral of two terms, one constant and one proportional to mean arterial blood-pressure. (Compare with the IPFM model of pacemaker control discussed earlier.)

Scher and Young (1963) found that the relationship between peripheral resistance and mean arterial blood-pressure consists of two sections, one frequency-dependent and one amplitude-dependent, apparently in cascade. We used the error function curve to describe the non-linearity, since only one parameter, sigma, is needed to specify shape. The relative positions of the sections were determined by attempting to simulate the spontaneous blood-pressure oscillations described earlier, which Stegmann and Giesen (1966) contended are a result of instability of the 'peripheral resistance reflex'. Fig. 10.14 is a simplified version of the peripheral resistance reflex. Initially, the configuration was as shown, with peripheral resistance, R_s, at the output from the non-linear element. As shown in the lower panel, however, even the smallest sustained oscillations in blood-pressure that could be simulated in the cardio-vascular model were 40 mm Hg, far larger than in the normal man. However, reversing the positions of the linear and non-linear sections (Fig. 10.15) produced oscillations comparable to those in healthy man, even with sigma at zero, where the non-linearity corresponds to an on–off element. As already discussed, the afferent/efferent brainstem interface of the peripheral resistance reflex is the likely site of the predicted on–off element; and the slow response of smooth muscle to neural stimulation, the low-pass filter.

Fig. 10.16 depicts Bevegard's finding (Bevegard, Holmgren, and Jonsson 1960) that, during orthostasis, mild exercise causes an almost 50 per cent increase in stroke volume and little change in heart-rate; whereas increases in workload increases the heart-rate but hardly affect stroke volume. Since both arteriolar resistance and venous capacitance vessels are innervated by similar sympathetic fibres, the same, highly non-linear, afferent/efferent interface probably also serves the 'venomotor tone reflex'. Dynamics of this reflex were obtained from Bartelstone's (1960) results. With regard to the 'left ventricular contractility reflex', simulation studies with the entire system model indicated this reflex to be more involved in myocardial energetics than in blood-pressure regulation, and for this reason it was omitted from the present simulation.

In Fig. 10.17, the reflex models are incorporated, orthostasis assumed,

205

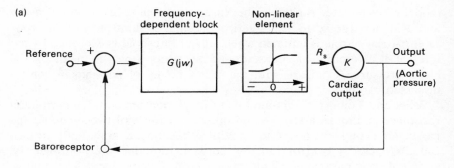

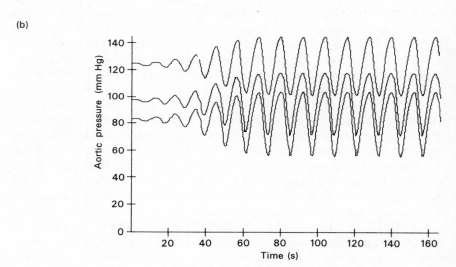

FIG. 10.14. (a) Highly simplified representation of the peripheral resistance reflex, showing the separately determined dynamic and static portions of the reflex; (b) spontaneous oscillations resulting from the configuration shown in (a).

and exercise is simulated by decreasing the metabolic component of peripheral resistance. As in man, the first 45 per cent increase in cardiac output is due to increase in stroke volume alone, and above that, to increase in heart-rate alone. Although the model is considerably more complex than the simple servo-mechanism, it nonetheless exhibits FSE (Fig. 10.18(c) and (d)). The hydraulic effect of respiration was simulated

206

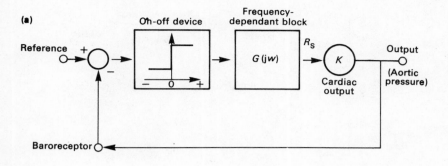

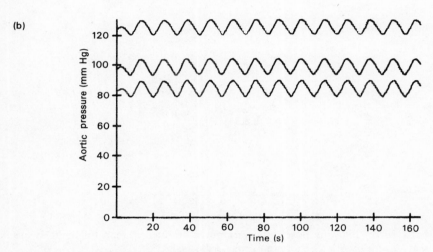

FIG. 10.15. (a) Highly simplified representation of the peripheral resistance reflex arranged as an on–off control system; (b) spontaneous oscillations resulting from the configuration shown in (a).

in the model by varying the simulated intrathoracic pressure in a sinusoidal manner. As in the physiological situation, the disturbance was chosen to be symmetrical about the resting expiratory value of intrathoracic pressure and the magnitude of the simulated disturbance was set equal to that observed in the experiment. That both the physiological system and the model thereof exhibit FSE provides further support that the model characterizes the important features of baroreceptor reflexes.

207

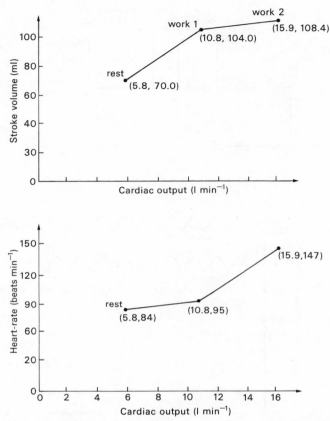

FIG. 10.16. Showing how cardiac output is attained in man for 'mild' (work 1) and 'severe' (work 2) exercise during orthostasis.

10.4. Cardiovascular disturbances of psychological origin

The aim of the most recent study (Hyndman 1976) was to determine whether the analysis technique described earlier could detect any changes persisting in the cardiac event sequence for a substantial period of time following a short but intense cognitive task and, if so, whether such changes could be identified with a particular physiological regulatory process.

The experiment was divided into nine sessions, A to I, corresponding sequentially to two pre-task rest sessions (A and B), one task session

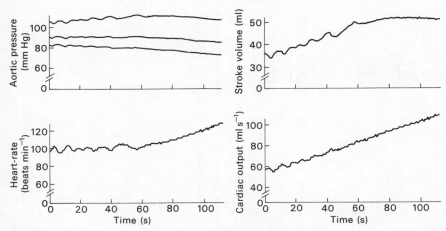

FIG. 10.17. Simulated exercise during orthostasis. Increases in cardiac output are achieved initially by increases in stroke volume alone and thereafter by increases in heart-rate alone.

(C), and six post-task rest sessions (D to I). Start-to-start session time was 10 min, except C–D and D–E which were 6 and 8 min, respectively. The time intervals between successive R wave maxima, obtained by electronic event detection of the ECG recordings of each session, were sampled from the start of each session for a duration of 3 min. Data was analysed from 21 separate experiments on 13 paid university student volunteers (8 of whom repeated the experiment 1 month later) who were screened by a routine medical examination.

The task duration was 3 min and consisted of the discrimination between two tones, 2000 Hz (high) and 500 Hz (low), generated in random sequence by a binary-choice generator. Each subject was instructed to respond to the high and low tones by pressing a microswitch with his right and left index finger, respectively. Earphones presented the tone binaurally at a fixed rate set to the maximum that the subject could answer with less than 2 errors per min for 3 min, as determined in a training session a few hours earlier (100 per cent binary choice task).

Fig. 10.19 displays for each experimental session the relative power distribution (the power of 0·05-Hz-wide spectral bands expressed as a fraction of the total spectral power) of the filtered cardiac event sequence (mean and linear trend removed). Each band corresponds to seven adjacent power spectrum coefficients obtained by the fast Fourier transform algorithm (Cooley and Tukey 1965) implemented on a Digital

209

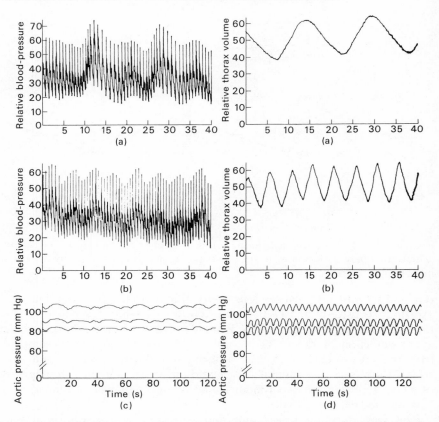

Fig. 10.18. 'Frequency-selective entrainment' in a normal man (a and b) and the model (c and d). (a) Two components in the blood-pressure, one of which has the same period (20 s) as voluntary respiration; (b) only one component, which also has the same period (5 s) as voluntary respiration; (c and d) behaviour in the model is the same as that in the man.

Equipment Corp. PDP-8/1 laboratory computer. Normalizing with respect to total power considerably reduces intersubject variance, possibly due to intersubject differences in pacemaker response to blood-pressure oscillations resulting from the effect of heart-rate on refractory period. The task can be seen to produce a large increase in the low-frequency content in session C, and the power in band 5 (the respiratory range during rest) shifts to band 6. Mean heart-rate was found to increase by 14 per cent ($p < 0.001$). With the completion of the task, the pre-task levels

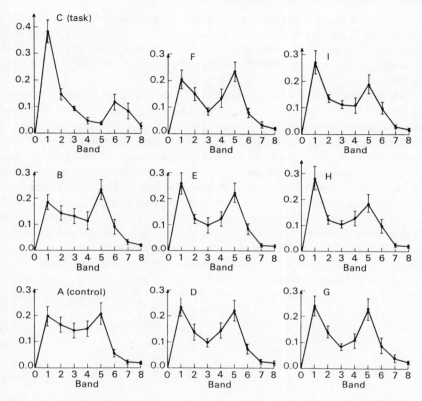

FIG. 10.19. The relative power distribution (±SE) of 0·05-Hz-wide spectral bands of the filtered cardiac event sequence. The panels correspond sequentially to two pre-task rest sessions (A and B), one task session (C), and six post-task sessions (D to I). Session duration is 10 min, except C and D which are 6 and 8 min, respectively. The task was a 100 per cent binary-choice task of 3-min duration.

(including heart-rate) are re-established in all but band 3 by the first post-task session (D). The depression in band 3 relative power apparent in sessions D, E, F, and G, persists until session H when it finally returns to its pre-task level, 43 min after task completion, at which time the over-all pre-task relative power distribution is thereby re-established.

It can be seen from these results that the persisting effect of the task is unlikely to be due to any variations in baroreflex gain since only one band is affected. Neither is it likely to be due to any respiratory entrainment

211

phenomenon as the respiratory components immediately return to pre-task levels. A more probable explanation is the persistence of some slow disturbance which thus alters the time-on to time-off ratio of the blood-pressure control system, thereby decreasing spontaneous oscillation magnitude.

This phenomenon is more compactly depicted in Fig. 10.20 by displaying band 3 relative power as a function of experimental session. In actual fact, the spectral range covered by bands 2, 3, and 4 of the entire set of 21 experiments was scanned to determine the exact frequency range where the most persisting post-task changes occurred. This range proved to have the same bandwidth as the original band 3, and the spectral limits are only one Fourier component (0·008 Hz) lower. Fig. 10.20 therefore represents the relative power in this slightly shifted band 3, which can be seen to decrease to half its pre-task value ($p < 0·01$) approximately 13 min after the task, and to remain significantly below the control value ($p < 0·05$) until session H, 43 min after the task completion.

Band 3 corresponds to spectral components of period between 10 and 7 s, the frequency range associated with blood-pressure homeostasis referred to earlier. That this regulating activity is depressed for such a

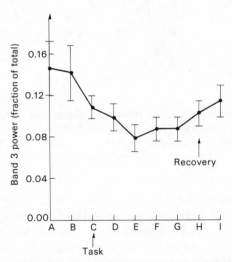

FIG. 10.20. Relative power (±SE) of the 7–10-s band of the filtered cardiac event sequence as a function of experimental session. This spectral range was found to display the most persisting post-task changes and corresponds to the frequency range associated with blood-pressure homeostasis.

substantial period of time following the short task suggests the involvement of task-activated and persisting hormone increases, such as circulating adrenalin, as reported by Johansson and Frankenhaüser (1973). As Levi (1971) has pointed out, the neuroendocrine reactions can influence nearly all physiological variables. Moreover, adrenalin has frequently been implicated in the pathogenesis of essential hypertension (Cuche, Kuchol, Barbeau, Langlois, Boucher, and Genest 1974; Saavedra, Grobecker, and Axelrod 1976; Brod 1971). However, the ability to raise adrenalin secretion during mental work has also been shown to be positively related to performance (Johansson and Frankenhaüser 1973). The subjects could be separated into two groups—those whose adrenalin returned rapidly to control values and those whose adrenalin recovery was much slower—and the faster group performed significantly better on the task and scored lower in a neuroticism personality test. These workers suggested that a slower recovery of adrenalin means either that the organism keeps secreting adrenalin when it is no longer required, or that it is less efficient in biochemically dissipating the substance, either of which is indicative of poor adjustment. As they put it, 'It is reasonable to assume that the rate at which adrenaline secretion returns to baseline levels after the cessation of the stressor may determine the relative potency of harmful and beneficial adrenaline effects'.

Brod's (1971) theory of stress-induced hypertension, in which the frequent mobilization of the defence response produces a protracted and eventually chronic blood-pressure elevation (as can be observed experimentally in animals), suggests that individuals with abnormally long recovery periods to a standard cognitive task might be more inclined to develop hypertension, particularly if they are frequently required to cope with situations which for them are mentally demanding. As Brod put it 'a new blood pressure rise may be started by another stimulus before the previous one has subsided completely. The pressor reactions would then eventually fuse'. Indeed, Brod (1963) and Baumann, Ziprian, Gödicke, Hartrodt, Naumann, and Laüter (1973) found that early hypertensives display a much more protracted recovery following a cognitive task than normotensives. The latter group attributed this protracted recovery to uneconomic biochemical reactions since a number of biochemical parameters displayed a similar prolonged task recovery.

It is interesting to note that similar personality characteristics are associated with individuals who exhibit slower physiological recovery after psychological effort (Johansson and Frankenhaüser 1973; Katkin 1966; Freeman 1939) and individuals who develop essential hypertension

(Brod 1971; Benson and Gutmann 1974; Richter-Heinrich and Laüter 1969; Weiner 1974). The suggestion that anxious or neurotic people may have little opportunity to recover from the constant stream of stimulation characteristic of contemporary life (Malmo 1957) may be the clue relating personality, recovery, and hypertension. As Malmo (1957) pointed out, slow recovery may be due to an inherited deficiency in certain physiological inhibitory mechanisms and/or a weakening of such mechanisms due to an individual constantly operating at physiological levels which are higher than normal. The obvious connection between personality and hypertension susceptibility has prompted Baumann to refer to this illness as a 'cerebrovisceral regulation disease' in which the pathogenic efficiency of stress depends largely on personality structure and stress sensitivity.

Evidence suggesting that hypertensives have overactive of even fused defence reactions can be interpreted from the results of Takeshita, Tanaka, Kuroiwa, and Nakamara (1975), who found that hypertensives have significantly lower baroreflex gain in heart-rate control. These workers ascribed such a gain reduction to changes in the central nervous system. The reduction in heart-rate variability with mental load (Hyndman and Gregory 1975) could also be a result of this gain reduction. Djojosugito, Folkow, Kylstra, Lisander, and Tuttle (1970) found such gain decreases to be a major feature of the defence reaction, by which hypothalamically-activated increases in heart-rate are not diminished by reflex inhibition via the baroreflex. Conversely, Smyth, Sleight, and Pickering (1969) have found baroreflex gain to be markedly enhanced during sleep.

Certain occupations accompanied by frequent exposure to mental stress, by an overload of responsibility, by frequent conflicting situations, are more frequently associated with hypertension, e.g., air traffic controllers, telephone operators. On the other hand, hypertension is less prevalent in people whose work involves heavy physical labour. This occupational difference in the incidence of hypertension may well be a result of the discoordination of the defence reflex discussed by Gilmore (1974) in which the hormonally produced changes of the blood are not dissipated in the normal way by a concomitant increase in metabolism.

There are apparently two systems acting to control human blood-pressure, viz., the baroreflex (neurogenic) and the fluid balance system of the kidney (Birkenhäger and Schalekamp 1976). Episodes of stress-induced blood-pressure elevation may well be neurogenically mediated but, in some manner, their repeated occurrence induces a sustained pressure which is not necessarily neurally mediated. Indeed, most experimental evidence favours the view that the role of the baroreflex is to buffer short-term changes of pressure but that over the long term they exert a permissive role by virtue of their resetting (adaptation). This short-term blood-pressure control appears then to act as a protective mechanism for the long-term pressure control system (kidney). However, activation of the defence reflex can override the baroreflex, as already discussed, for the purpose of providing the body with the critical means to take defensive physical action. If the resulting increase in blood-pressure is prolonged, as a result of the associated release of hormones into the blood remaining undissipated due to insufficient metabolic activity or a malfunctioning of biochemical inhibitory mechanisms, the result may be damage to the kidney ultrastructure. Indeed, renal vascular resistance has been reported to increase with advancing hypertension (Birkenhäger and Schalekamp 1976). This need only be slightly out of proportion to the over-all resistance increase to cancel the effects of an increased blood-pressure on fluid excretion. As a result of the action of whole body auto-regulation, the resulting increase in cardiac output will be returned to normal by the widespread constriction of the resistance vessels (substantiated by the reported progressive non-autonomic reduction in vascular calibre (Birkenhäger and Schalekamp 1976)). As a result, the arterial pressure will be sustained at a higher than normal value.

Even before chronic elevation in blood-pressure sets in, long-recovery individuals exposed to an environment comprising any particular sequence of psychological stimuli would evidence a greater mean blood-pressure elevation—possibly to the extent of damaging the kidney ultrastructure—over the period of exposure, and thus load on the heart as well, than would normal recovery individuals exposed to the same environment. Frequent prolonged episodes of elevated blood-pressure or circulating catecholamine concentration may have consequences to kidney function (Weiner 1974; Birkenhäger and Schalekamp 1976), and thus ultimately to long-term blood-pressure homeostasis (Guyton, Coleman, Bower, and Granger 1970). Indeed, Birkenhäger (1976) has found such pronounced stress-induced blood-pressure elevations to be associated with higher mean values of blood-pressure months after the stressful episode.

In addition to the possible clinical usefulness of the recovery phenomenon as a dynamic test for susceptibility to stress-induced hypertension, scaling a frequently repeated and mentally demanding occupational task according to the average time required for recovery may give a relative indication of the task's potential hazard to health. In this connection, significant individual deviations could reveal particular aptitude and/or attitude anomalies for that task, assuming normal recovery to the standard (neutral) task. Moreover, such an approach would not only provide a quantative basis for task restructuring (to ensure the assignment of adequate recovery time to particularly demanding tasks) but would also make it possible to assess the efficiency (in terms of reducing physiological recovery time) of various recreational activities during 'rest' phases.

10.5. Non-invasive blood-pressure measurement

Up to this point we have had to be content with some measure of 'activity' of the blood-pressure control system by way of a rather elaborate signal processing of the electrocardiogram, this being one of the few available reliable non-invasive cardiovascular measurements. However, in 1973 an instrument was reported at the 10th International Conference on Medical and Biological Engineering in Dresden, G.D.R., for the non-invasive continuous measurement of human arterial blood-pressure (Penaz 1973). An instrument patterned closely along the lines of that first prototype, and incorporating a number of important improvements, has been developed for the Netherlands Institute for Preventive Medicine, TNO, Leiden, at the Institute for Medical Physics, TNO, Utrecht, the Netherlands (Hyndman, Snoeck, Wesseling, and de Wit 1978).

The instrument follows the method of Penaz (1973, 1976), using the principle of the unloaded vascular wall. A transducer comprising a photoelectric plethysmograph and inflatable cuff is fitted to the finger. The plethysmographic signal is used to operate an air valve which controls the pressure in the cuff so that the plethysmographic signal is clamped to a pre-set value. If this value is made to correspond to the unloaded region of the finger arteries diameter, the cuff pressure will follow the instantaneous pressure in those arteries. The choice of photo-plethysmography over other forms has the advantage that the signal obtained is sensitive only to changes in blood volume and not to changes in extravascular fluid volumes which ensue when external pressure is applied to an extremity.

The instrument, including finger cuff, is shown in Fig. 10.21. The development comprises four separate problems, viz., the design and construction of the finger cuff, the design and construction of the fast-acting air valve, the electronic compensation of the feedback control system in order to achieve accurate stable clamping of the plethysmogram

216

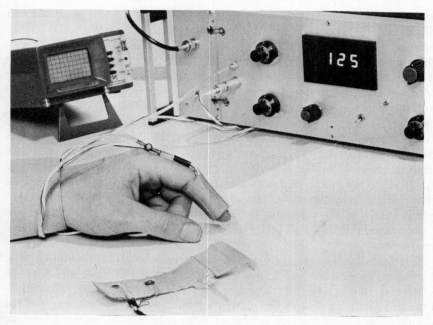

FIG. 10.21. The instrument, comprising the finger cuff (in which the photocells can be seen) and the unit containing the electronics and electrically driven air valve. Beat-to-beat systolic, diastolic, or mean blood-pressure can be displayed, as well as a continuous registration. The oscilloscope is used to determine the plethysmogram reference level.

to the reference level, and the development of a procedure for the adjustment of the reference level.

The design of the cuff is determined by the following considerations. The cuff volume should be kept minimal as this is the major factor affecting the dynamic performance of the instrument. The cuff length is determined by the longtitudinal distribution of pressure transmitted from the cuff to the arterial wall (Steinfeld, Alexander, and Cohen 1974), as well as the light source–sensor field pattern. The cuff material must be thin enough for distortionless pressure transmission to the finger but strong enough to support the whole arterial pressure at the cuff ends. The photoelectric source–sensor pair must generate as little heat as possible, be insensitive to blood oxygen changes (Lee, Tahmoush, and Jennings 1975), be compact enough to fit in a small cuff, and have a dynamic response exceeding 50 Hz, this being more than adequate to follow the

217

arterial blood-pressure waveform. As can be seen from Fig. 10.21 our finger cuff is virtually a miniaturized version of the conventional sphygmomanometer cuff; the photoelectric diodes come into direct contact with the finger. This cuff has a number of advantages over the Penaz unit which comprises a number of inflatable plastic sacks inside a rigid cylinder with light source and sensor mounted in the cylinder such that the light must pass through the sacks as well as the finger. Owing to the direct skin contact, a much larger plethysmogram can be obtained with our type of cuff. Motion artefact is substantially reduced also as a result of this intimate contact with the finger plus the absence of the inertia (and thus motion relative to the finger) of a rigid cylinder. Our unit fits a large range of finger sizes. With this cuff design, the air volume is minimized (approximately 1 ml), this being the major determinant of the dynamic performance of the instrument. Finally, the cuff is disposable (the photocells are removable) and unobtrusive and thus suitable for clinical environments.

The fast-acting electrically driven air valve follows the technique used by Penaz in which a small loudspeaker provides the basic structure. A small flat metal plate is fastened to the spider of the loudspeaker and a nozzle is mounted against the plate in such a way that displacement of the speaker cone controls the amount of air which can escape from the nozzle. The nozzle is connected to a T-junction, one leg of which is a flow constriction connected to a compressed air source, the other the inflatable cuff. This 'controlled leak' has dynamic properties which can be compensated for in the electronics of the instrument to allow accurate stable clamping of the plethysmogram to the reference level.

The reference level to which the plethysmogram is clamped is determined by the following procedure. The feedback loop is opened, i.e. the plethysmogram is disconnected from the air valve and displayed on an oscilloscope, and the cuff pressure is adjusted externally until the plethysmogram pulsations are maximal, the reference level adjusted to the d.c. value of the plethysmogram, and the loop again closed. It can be shown that the diameter of the finger arteries will now be maintained at a value corresponding to their unloaded region (zero transmural pressure). Fig. 10.22 illustrates that when the loop is closed (arrow), any deviations in vascular volume due to changes in intravascular pressure are immediately compensated by adjustment of cuff pressure which therefore follows the intravascular pressure waveform. The shape of the cuff pressure waveform is highly similar to directly-recorded, peripheral blood-pressure (Eggink 1959).

218

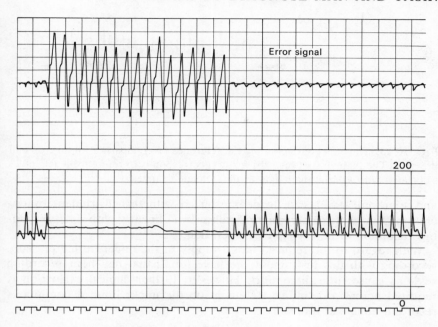

FIG. 10.22. Showing how the instrument 'clamps' the plethysmogram to a fixed value by producing a pressure cuff waveform equal to that in the finger arteries.

As a first evaluation, we compared systolic and diastolic values obtained with the instrument with the corresponding values obtained from conventional sphygmamanometry on the contralateral arm in ten subjects, taking care that the finger was positioned at heart level. The mean values of systolic and diastolic pressure did not differ significantly between the methods ($p < 0.2$), the mean error being approximately 10 mm Hg. Of course, sphygmomanometry is itself subject to error (Van Bergen, Weatherhead, Treloar, Dobkin, and Buckley 1954) and the most desirable comparison would be to direct intra-arterial measurements; only then can an assessment of true measurement error be made. This is planned in the near future. Preliminary results (7 patients) of such a study show a discrepancy of only a few per cent between the arterial pressure measured directly in the brachial artery and that obtained non-invasively with this instrument (Wesseling 1978).

Fig. 10.23 shows that the plateau in the arterial pressure–volume relationship, characteristic of the unstressed region of an artery (Vendrik

219

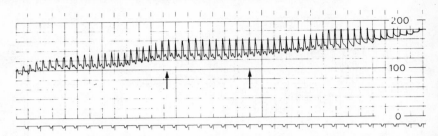

FIG. 10.23. The effect of decreasing the reference level linearly with time on cuff pressure. The plateau (between the arrows) corresponds to reference level values associated with arterial diameters in the unloaded range.

and Vierhout 1959), can be demonstrated with this instrument by decreasing the plethysmographic reference level linearly with time, providing validation of its principle of operation.

With regard to the reduced blood-supply to the finger during pressure recording with this instrument, we have found that half-hour recording sessions cause little discomfort. However, further clinical evaluation is required before a definitive statement on the upper limit of continuous recording time can be made.

10.6. Analysis of the arterial blood-pressure signal

With access to the arterial blood-pressure signal, a number of studies are now possible. To name a few:

(a) Comparison of mean blood-pressure recovery to a defined psychological task in normotensives and early hypertensives; follow-up studies to determine whether recovery time is a reliable predictor of hypertension.

(b) Comparison of mean blood-pressure recovery in normotensives to psychological tasks of differing complexities; is recovery time determined by task complexity? Intra- and inter-occupational comparison of task recovery time.

(c) Comparison of mean blood-pressure recovery in normotensives to a defined psychological task followed by a rest period and by a defined physical task. Does the physical task alter recovery to the psychological task?

(d) Comparison of mean blood-pressure recovery in normotensives to a defined psychological task when insufficient time is given to allow complete recovery to a preceding task. Is carry-over evident?

(e) Comparison of mean blood-pressure recovery curve in normotensives to a standard psychological task with simultaneously obtained recovery curve of circulating adrenalin, to establish the physiological basis of the recovery phenomenon.

Other applications are numerous, e.g. inclusion of blood-pressure recording during psychiatric interviews to determine stressful life situations for patients (Groen, Hansen, Hermann, Schäfer, Schmidt, Selbmann, Uexküll, and Wechmann 1977), in biofeedback and autogenic configurations to treat hypertension, in testing the efficacy of hypotensive drugs, etc.

Moreover, in order to study the operation of the blood-pressure regulatory system, it is now possible to investigate the spectral content of the blood-pressure signal in man under various circumstances. For example, Bagshaw, Fronek, Peterson, and Zinsser (1975) have found that hypertensives do not display the 10-s periodicity associated with blood-pressure homeostasis found in normal man (Hyndman 1974). Baroreflex sensitivity, another important parameter of the blood-pressure regulatory system (Takeshita *et al.* 1975; Smyth *et al.* 1969) can now also be estimated non-invasively by comparing the spectrum of the cardiac event sequence, obtained as discussed earlier, with that of the (non-invasively recorded) blood-pressure signal.

With regard to the 10-s blood-pressure component, further evidence of its importance has been found by Szücs, Monos, and Csaki (1975). Using dogs, they found that after experimental haemorrhage, although mean blood-pressure could be restored by re-infusion, the 10-s component did not return, indicative of irreversible damage to the baroreflex, and the dogs died soon after. Perhaps a running spectral display of the blood-pressure signal may, in the future, prove to be of greater value to the anaesthetist, as an indication of the 'state' of cardiovascular homeostasis, than of mean blood-pressure. Further studies are clearly warranted.

References

BAGSHAW, R. J., FRONEK, A., PETERSON, L. H., and ZINSSER, H. F. (1975). Dispersion of blood pressure and heart rate in essential hypertension. *IEEE Trans. Bio-med. Engng (Inst. elect. electron. Engrs)* **22,** 508–12.

BARTELSTONE, H. J. (1960). Role of the veins in venous return, *Circulation Res.* **8,** 1059–76.

BAUMANN, R., ZIPRIAN, H., GÖDICKE, W., HARTRODT, W., NAUMANN, E., and LAÜTER, J. (1973). The influence of acute psychic stress situations on biochemical and vegetative parameters of essential hypertensives at the early stage of the disease. *J. Psychother. Psychosom.* **22,** 131–40.

BAYLEY, E. J. (1968). Spectral analysis of pulse frequency modulation in the nervous system. *IEEE Trans. Bio-med. Engng* (*Inst. elect. electron. Engrs*) **15**, 257–65.

BENEKEN, J. E. W. (1965). A mathematical approach to cardiovascular function. Ph.D. dissertation, Institute for Medical Physics, Utrecht, TNO.

BENSON, H. and GUTMANN, M. C. (1974). The relation of environmental factors to systemic arterial hypertension. In *Stress and the heart* (ed. R. S. Eliot), pp. 13–31. Futura, New York.

BEVEGARD, S., HOLMGREN, A., and JONSSON, B. (1960). The effect of body position on the circulation at rest and during exercise, with special reference to the influence on the stroke volume. *Acta Physiol. scand.* **49**, 279–98.

BIRKENHÄGER, W. H. (1976). Inaugural Lecture, Erasmus University, Rotterdam.

—— and SCHALEKAMP, M. A. D. H. (1976). *Control mechanisms in essential hypertension.* Elsevier, Amsterdam.

BROD, J. (1963). Hemodynamic basis of acute pressor reactions and hypertension. *Br. Heart J.* **19**, 227–45.

—— (1971). The influence of higher nervous processes induced by psychosocial environment on the development of essential hypertension. In *Society, stress and disease* (ed. L. Levi), Vol. 1. Oxford University Press, London.

COOLEY, J. W. and TUKEY, J. W. (1965). An algorithm for the machine calculation of complex Fourier series. *Math. Comput.* **19**, 297–301.

CUCHE, J. L., KUCHEL, O., BARBEAU, A., LANGLOIS, Y., BOUCHER, R., and GENEST, J. (1974). Autonomic nervous system and benign essential hypertension in man. *Circulation Res.* **35**, 281–9.

DJOJOSUGITO, A. M., FOLKOW, B., KYLSTRA, P. H., LISANDER, B., and TUTTLE, R. S. (1970). Differentiated intersections between the hypothalmic defence reaction and baroreceptor reflexes. 1. Effects on heart rate and regional flow resistance, *Acta Physiol. Scand.* **78**, 376–85.

EGGINK, A. A. (1959). De betekenis van de arteriële en veneuze pulsatiecurven voor de diagnostiek van aangeboren hartgebreken. Ph.D. thesis, University of Amsterdam.

FREEMAN, G. L. (1939). Toward a psychological plimsoll mark: physiological recovery quotients in experimentally induced frustration. *J. Psychol.* **8**, 247–52.

GILMORE, J. P. (1974). Physiology of stress. In *Stress and the heart* (ed. R. S. Eliot), pp. 69–90. Futura, New York.

GROEN, J. J., HANSEN, B., HERMANN, J. M., SCHÄFER, N., SCHMIDT, T. H., SELBMANN, K. H., UEXKÜLL, T. V., and WECHMANN, P. (1977). Haemodynamic responses during experimental emotional states and physical exercise in hypertensive and normotensive patients. In *Hypertension and brain mechanisms* (eds W. de Jong and A. P. Provost), pp. 301–8. Elsevier, Amsterdam.

GUYTON, A. C., COLEMAN, T. G., BOWER, J. D., and GRANGER, H. J. (1970). Circulatory control in hypertension, *Circulation Res.* (*Suppl. 2*) 135–47.

HYNDMAN, B. W. (1973). An example of digital computer simulation: investigation of the human cardiovascular system. In *Computer techniques in biomedicine and medicine* (ed. E. Haga), pp. 98–120. Auerbach, Philadelphia.

—— (1974). The role of rhythms in homeostasis. *Kybernetik* **15,** 227–36.

—— (1976). Signal analysis and modeling in psychophysiology research. In *Digest of the 11th International Conference on Medical and Biological Engineering,* Ottawa, pp. 194–5.

—— and GREGORY, J. R. (1975). Spectral analysis of sinus arrhythmia during mental loading. *Ergonomics* **18,** 255–70.

—— and MOHN, R. K. (1975). A model of the cardiac pacemaker and its use in decoding the information content of cardiac intervals. *Automed.* **1,** 239–52.

——, SNOECK, B., WESSELING, K. H., and DE WIT, B. (1978). An instrument for the noninvasive continuous measurement of absolute arterial blood pressure, *Proceedings of the 3rd International Conference on Cardiovascular System Dynamics, Leiden* (eds J. Baan and A. C. Arntzenius), p. 21. Excerpta Medica, Amsterdam.

JOHANSSON, G. and FRANKENHAUSER, M. (1973). Temporal factors in sympatho-adrenomedullary activity following acute behavioral activation. *Biol. Psych.* **1,** 63–73.

KATKIN, E. (1966). The relationship between a measure of transitory anxiety and spontaneous autonomic activity, *J. abnorm. Psychol.* **71,** 142–6.

LEE, A. L., TAHMOUSH, A. J., and JENNINGS, J. R. (1975). An LED-transistor photoplethysmograph. *IEEE Trans. Bio-med. Engng (Inst. elect. electron. Engrs)* **22,** 248–50.

LEVI, L. (Ed.) (1971). *Society, stress and disease,* Vol. 1. Oxford University Press, London.

MALMO, R. B. (1957). Anxiety and behavioral arousal. *Psychol. Rev.* **64,** 276–87.

PENAZ, J. (1973). Photoelectric measurement of blood pressure, volume and flow in the finger. In *Digest of the 10th International Conference on Medical and Biological Engineering,* p. 104. Dresden.

—— (1976). Beitrag zur fortlaufenden indirekten Blutdrukmessung. *Z. gesam. innere Med. Grenzgebiete* **31,** 1030–3.

RICHTER-HEINRICH, E. and LAÜTER, J. (1969). A psychophysiological test as diagnostic tool with essential hypertensives. *Psychother. Psychosom.* **17,** 153–68.

SAAVEDRA, J. M., GROBECKER, H., and AXELROD, J. (1976). Adrenaline-forming enzyme in brainstem: elevation in genetic and experimental hypertension. *Science* **191,** 483–4.

SCHER, A. M. and YOUNG, A. C. (1963). Servoanalysis of carotid sinus reflex effects on peripheral resistance. *Circulation Res.* **17,** 152–62.

SMYTH, H. S., SLEIGHT, P., and PICKERING, G. W. (1969). Reflex regulation of arterial pressure during sleep in man. *Circulation Res.* **24,** 109–21.

SNYDER, M. F. and RIDEOUT, V. C. (1969). Computer simulation studies of the venous circulation, *IEEE Trans. bio-med. Engng (Inst. elect. electron. Engrs)* **16,** 325–34.

STEGEMANN, J. and GEISEN, K. (1966). Zur regeltheoretischen Analyse des Blutkreislaufes. *Pflüger's Arch. ges. Physiol.* **287,** 276–85.

STEINFELD, L., ALEXANDER, H., and COHEN, M. L. (1974). Updating sphygmomanometry. *Amer. J. Cardiol.* **33,** 107–10.

SZÜCS, B., MONOS, E., and CSAKI, F. (1975). New aspects of blood pressure control. In *Digest 6th Triennial World Congress of International Federation of Automatic Control,* Cambridge, Mass.

TAKESHITA, A., TANAKA, S., KUROIWA, A., and NAKAMURA, M. (1975). Reduced baroreceptor sensitivity in borderline hypertension. *Circulation* **31,** 738–42.

VAN BERGEN, F. H., WEATHERHEAD, D. S., TRELOAR, A. E., DOBKIN, A. B., and BUCKLEY, J. J. (1954). Comparison of indirect and direct methods of measuring arterial blood pressure. *Circulation* **10,** 481–90.

VENDRIK, A. J. H. and VIERHOUT, R. R. (1959). Die unblutige Registrierung des Blutdruks. Theoretische Betrachtungen *Pflüger's Arch. ges. Physiol.* **268,** 496–509.

WAGNER, R. (1950). Die Regulierung des Blutdruckes als Beispiel einer Regler-Einrichtung im Organismus. *Naturwiss.* **37,** 128–36.

WEIDINGER, H., HETZEL, R., and SCHAEFER, H. (1962). Aktionsströme in zentrifugalen vagalen Herznerven und deren Bedeutung für den Kreislauf. *Pflüger's Arch. ges. Physiol.* **276,** 262–79.

WEINER, H. (1974). Psychosomatic research in essential hypertension: retrospect and prospect. In *Stress and the heart* (ed. R. S. Eliot), pp. 58–116. Futura, New York.

WESSELING, K. H. (1978). Niet invasieve vinger-bloeddrukmeter, Boerhave Wetenschappelijk Rapport. *Afdeling Cardiologie, Leiden,* October 6, 1978.

11.
Heart-rate variability in psychiatry
R. E. OFFERHAUS

11.1. Introduction

HEART-RATE variability (HRV) or beat-to-beat variation has long been known to be correlated with respiration. Furthermore, it has been known to be affected by the psychic state. Wiersma (1913) noticed the great differences in heart frequency, pulse amplitude, and respiratory arrhythmia occurring at different psychical states or different degrees of 'consciousness'. The relation between heart-rate and its fluctuations and psychiatry has been investigated by a number of of authors (e.g. Sherman 1945; Berger 1964; Acker 1964; Crooks and McNulty 1966; Leder 1966; Kelly and Walter 1968; Kelly, Brown, and Schaffer 1970; Flekköy and Ashup 1969; Porges and Raskin 1969; Lader and Mattheus 1970; Fenz and Velner 1970; Miller and Bernal 1971; Varni, Clark, and Giddon 1971; Porges 1972, 1976; Walter and Porges 1976).

In recent work on HRV, no use is now made of any such ill-defined concept as 'consciousness', but the subject is placed into different sets of controlled and often quantitatively measurable conditions. The external stimulus then serves as the independent variable, with HRV and other physiological parameters as the dependent variables. The results of these studies are not always in agreement with each other. This is partly caused by the fact that HRV is measured differently by different workers. Furthermore, HRV reacts differently to different kinds of stimuli.

Thus, for example, Kalsbeek (1967) and Ettema (1967) analysed HRV over a period of minutes, with and without mental loading. Their aim was to determine the mental capacity for specific information tasks and the effect of such tasks on physiological parameters. They regard the 'psychic apparatus' as a processor of information. If this is a valid theoretical concept, it should be possible to analyse the capacity of this 'psychic apparatus' in handling different kinds of information, and to analyse inter-individual differences and moment-to-moment differences in capacity. To measure this capacity they offered the subject a binary choice task.

In a task of this kind they found HRV and respiration to be the best physiological parameters. Now, we have carried out a number of experiments using their method, to investigate whether it could be used with any reliability and validity in psychiatry. As the method is new, especially in psychiatry, we made an analysis on 5 different HRV variables, and conducted test—retest analyses and rest-mental task analyses. The experiments and the analyses, as well as the question of the validity of using HRV as a diagnostic tool in psychiatry, will be discussed.

11.2. Methods and procedures

For the information task, use was made of a binary-choice task. Subjects were presented with one stimulus out of a set of two and were asked to react by pressing the appropriate key out of two. As the two stimuli were offered in random order, it was impossible for the subjects to predict which stimulus would come next.

Sequences of more than 6 equal stimuli were eliminated, because this leads to faulty reactions with all subjects. This elimination was necessary to enable the subject to follow the instruction not to make any mistakes. In our programme we offered the stimuli at a fixed rate, instead of allowing the subject to determine his own speed by offering the next stimulus immediately after his reaction to the foregoing. As stimuli we chose red lamps fixed in a table in front of the subject. For keys we used finger-tip keys fixed on the same table in front of the lamps. Subjects were instructed to press the left key when the left lamp lit and the right key when the right lamp lit. This system requires hardly any motor effort. Moreover, it prevents feelings of isolation, which, compared with an earphone system, has advantages in a psychiatric institute. In this research use was made of precordial leads, an ECG amplifier and a hardware R wave detector. The digitally measured RR intervals are stored in a memory of a specially developed hardware system.

We did not assemble a histogram of the RR intervals, but a sequential curve (tachogram) (see Fig. 11.1). This curve was recorded on paper. If it showed no artefacts, the HRV variables computed from the intervals and fed into our hardware system, were accepted for further study. The HRV variables computed with the aid of this special purpose computer, are the following:

1. Heart rate (HR): number of RR intervals + 1 per 4 min.

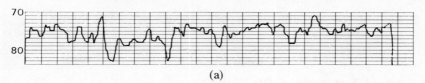

(a)

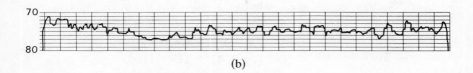

(b)

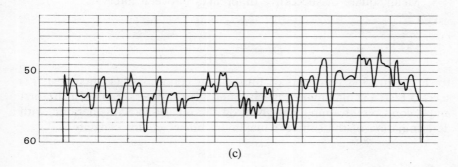

(c)

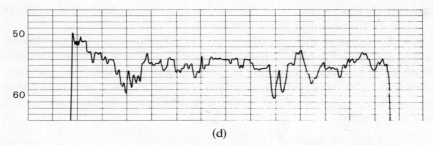

(d)

FIG. 11.1. Four examples of tachograms (four minutes): (a) member of staff; condition: rest (HR = 306, N = 164, S = 7437); (b) same member of staff; condition: binary choice task (HR = 319, N = 248, S = 7719); (c) patient; condition: rest (HR = 293, N = 116, S = 3881); (d) same patient; condition: binary choice task (HR = 308, N = 134, S = 2919).

227

2. Sum of absolute differences between successive RR intervals

$$S = \sum_{i=2}^{HR-1} |X_i - X_{i-1}|$$

where X_i = length of IBI 'i' in ms.

3. Number of fluctuations in the cardiotachogram:

$$N = Z \quad \text{where} \quad \begin{aligned} Z &= 1 \quad \text{if} \quad Y < 0 \\ Z &= 0 \quad \text{if} \quad Y > 0 \end{aligned}$$

$$Y = (X_i - X_{i-1})(X_{i-1} - X_{i-2})$$
$$(i = 3, 4, \dots, HR-1)$$

4. S/N

5. Mean square of successive differences between intervals:

$$D^2 = \frac{\sum_{i-1}^{HR-2} (X_{i-1} - X_i)^2}{HR-2}$$

Each registration consisted of four 4-min conditions: (1) first rest; (2) second rest; (3) maximum capacity; and (4) third rest. Between the first and second rest, training was given on the binary-choice generator, with determination of the subject's maximum binary-choice capacity

$$C_{mbc} = \hat{C} - a$$

where $\hat{C}$ is the maximum number of binary choices per minute when the subject is allowed to make no more than 7 errors or omissions and a is a constant chosen in order that the subject can sustain the task at C_{mbc}; in practice this constant is chosen to be 10.

All the subjects were members of the population of the psychiatric centre St. Bavo of which 211 patients and 72 staff members participated. A division was made between medicated and non-medicated patients. Furthermore psychological testing, biochemical analyses, and movement observations were carried out. Three measuring sessions took place, each two weeks apart.

11.3. Results

HRV *parameters*

Beat-to-beat variation, or as it is called now, heart-rate variability, is usually only based on several RR intervals. Most investigators compare some intervals before and some intervals following a certain stimulus. In our study, however, we continuously registered HRV and computed the above-mentioned variables. As we used a registration period of 4 min, we registered some 270 to 370 RR intervals from which the variables were computed. The registration was done under fixed and standardized conditions, of both rest and task. Some examples of registered interval sequences are shown in Fig. 11.1.

Four-minute measurements of heart-rate variability yield scores that show no differences from scores obtained two weeks before or two weeks afterwards with the same person, under the same conditions, the only differences in the scores being brought about by the condition applied, i.e. the mental task set to the subject. The method used, and especially the HR and HRV scoring technique, proves to be test—retest reliable. This is the more remarkable as 211 of the 283 subjects were psychiatric patients. In such a population one would expect an increased variability, with a certain proportion of the patients being variable in their 'psychic or autonomic state'. As stated, this variability did not appear in our test—retest analysis.

Apparently, a 4-min period is long enough to obviate unsystematic influences not relevant to the 'state' of a person, such as startle reactions, reactions to occasional sounds or light changes, or to thoughts occurring during rest conditions. Mulder and Mulder (1972), who developed the scoring methods we used, also found a 4-min period to be reliable, in the sense that if the stimulus task set remained unchanged, the HR and HRV scores of any 4-min period were not clearly different from those of another registration with the same person on another day. As we worked with a psychiatric population and were unable to fix visits on specific days and at a specific time during the day, a greater day-to-day variance could have been expected.

A detailed discussion of the results and the applied statistical analysis methods lies beyond the scope of this chapter. The interested reader is referred to Offerhaus (1977a, b). We used five different variables from the ECG. From the recorded tachograms of the ECG's the variables HR, N, S, S/N, and D^2 were computed. Factor analysis showed S, S/N, and D^2 contained the same information. Variables N and HR also correlated, but not so strongly as the first three. We decided to eliminate the variables S/N and D^2 from our further research because they are evidently redundant.

Of the three remaining HRV variables, HR and N show a distinct tendency to fall off during each test period of four conditions (Figs 11.1

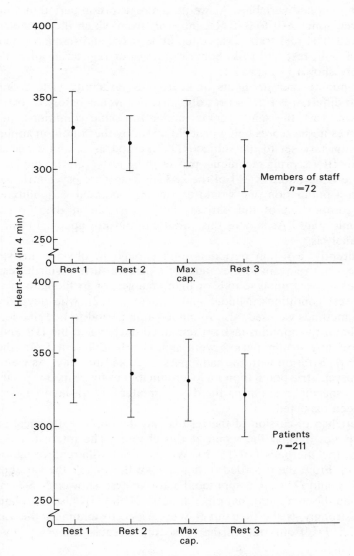

FIG. 11.2. Mean and standard deviation of HR in the four conditions, registered for members of staff and patients.

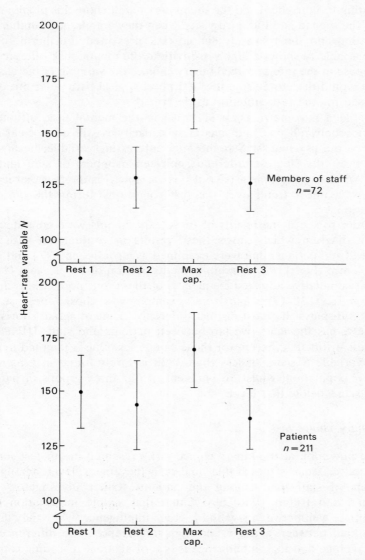

F IG. 11.3. Mean and standard deviation of N in the four conditions, registered for members of staff and patients.

and 11.3). As the whole test procedure takes up to an hour, there is apparently a gradual lowering of the arousal level of the subjects. It is interesting to note that even the members of staff show this phenomenon during the second and the third visits, when they are already familiar with the setting and the relatively simple task presented. Furthermore, the HRV variable N shows a high sensitivity to the mental task offered: with an increase in the rate of forced binary choices the variable N increases as well. It would therefore seem the best physiological parameter out of the ones used for the task situation as described.

Variable S is somewhat less sensitive to the mental task, although a difference between rest and maximum capacity is still quite clear (Fig. 11.4). To the psychiatrist S is the most interesting variable, because its scores show the clearest difference between members of staff and patients. Another noticeable aspect of this variable S is the fact that it does not show a linear trend over the rest conditions during the one-hour registration.

In order to see if the results of these experiments were consistent we made a diagram which shows these results in conjunction with data obtained from patients that were examined as a routine in 1974 and 1975 in our centre (Fig. 11.5). It exhibits the dispersion of 80 per cent (10–90 per cent cumulative adjusted frequency) of these four populations during condition 'rest 3'. (This particular example was chosen because this condition displays the most distinct differences.) The diagram shows that variable S has the least overlap between patients and staff, HR and N being less distinctly different for those categories. One is tempted to state that a variable S score of less than 3700 is rarely found in a mentally 'healthy' population, whilst 40 per cent of our three groups of patients have a score below that level.

The binary-choice task

If we now look at the binary choice task presented in our test setting, we found a clearly observable higher achievement level among the members of staff than among the patients. Other investigators (e.g. Friedman and Rubin 1966) also found that simple information tasks differentiate well between low and average intelligence, while they do not differentiate between average and high intelligence. The difference between average and high intelligence is one of abstract reasoning capacity rather than of information handling capacity.

As a large proportion of the patients in a psychiatric institute have a

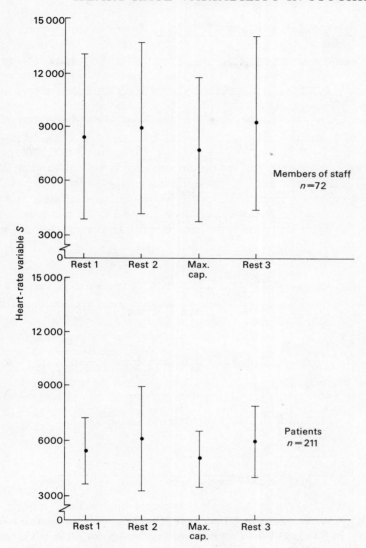

FIG. 11.4. Mean and standard deviation of S in the four conditions, registered for members of staff and patients.

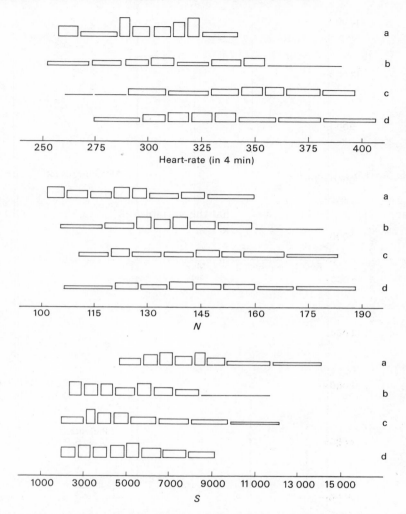

FIG. 11.5. The despersion of 80 per cent (10–90 per cent cumulative adjusted frequency) of four populations during condition 'rest 3' for three HRV parameters. (a) The members of staff; (b) the research patient population; (c) the patients registered on a routine basis in 1974 ($n = 110$); (d) the patients registered on a routine basis in 1975 ($n = 164$). Each rectangle represents 10 per cent of the population (the area of each rectangle is the same); (the 'lowest' 10 per cent and the 'highest' 10 per cent were disregarded in this figure.)

below-average intelligence (mentally retarded and/or psychotic) and trad-itional intelligence tests on such patients often give rise to problems, the binary-choice capacity measurements technique seems very suitable for use in such populations. This is all the more true because binary-choice capacity is easy to measure, can be repeated often without any great learning effect, and takes only 60 min. Another advantage is that patients like the procedure: they regard it as a sport rather than as a psychological test. They try to obtain the highest possible score and are keen to hear whether they did better than last time.

Influence of medication

A comparison of the patient groups with and without psychophar-macoligical medication showed that the variables HR and N only differed during the task condition and did not during rest. The variable S in the main study appeared to be independent of medication. However, in a separate study with subjects with anti-psychotic medication, condition 'rest 2' showed a difference for the medication group compared with a placebo group. Conditions 'rest 1' and 'rest 2' showed no differences. There are two ways of looking at these findings. On the one hand, one tends to be glad the measurement variable is not influenced, especially since it is a somatic parameter. On the other hand, it would have been very welcome if medication would have influenced heart-rate variability and patients would have attained a better condition. This is not the case.

Anti-psychotic medication seems to have a positive effect on the capacity, a higher binary choice capacity is reached when medication has an anti-psychotic effect, but neither in acute, nor in chronic patients does it affect the HRV variables in rest.

Relationship between psychological data and HRV findings

In an effort to give binary-choice capacity and the HRV variables a place in the nomological network of psychology, we performed several first- and second-order factor analyses on HRV-, psychological, and biochemical data. They yielded the three second-order factors that are often found by investigators, viz. capacity, extraversion, and anxiety. The last factor had the highest loadings in our population, which is not surprising because we did our experiments in a psychiatric centre. On this anxiety factor loadings were high for the clinical Minnesota Multiphasic Personality Inventory (MMPI) scales, like ego strength and schizophrenia, a catecholamine dopamine, and the heart variables HR, N, and S. On the

235

second or capacity factor high loadings were found for age, IQ, movement, and binary-choice capacity scores. The third factor was mainly determined by the social introversion scale of the MMPI, the extraversion scale of the Amsterdam Biographic Questionnaire (ABQ), and a specific urinary biochemical component (5-HIAA).

Possible groupings on the basis of HRV parameters

The last problem we wanted to investigate was: can the HRV variables be used as a separation criterion between groups? First of all, there is of course the question whether there are any subdivisions to make in the population studied on the basis of these variables. Friedman and Rubin cluster analysis showed that with a reasonably high probability there are four groups in the population. These 4 groups were analysed and compared with each other. One staff group can be characterized as 'highly normal': they have average age, capacity, HRV variables, and low lie, anxiety, and neuroticism scores. The other staff group can be characterized as 'neurotic': they have average age, capacity, and HRV variables N and S' and low lie and anxiety scores, but their heart-rate is high, mean 88·5 per minute, and their neuroticism scores are somewhat on the high side.

The first patient group is the 'chronic' group: they are older, have a low capacity, low neuroticism scores, an average HR and HRV variable N, but a low HRV variable S score and high lie and anxiety scores. The second patient group is a mixture of chronic and acute patients, but the latter dominate. So it should be described as the 'acute' group: average age, but low capacity, high lie, anxiety, and neuroticism scores; a very high HR and HRV variable N and a low HRV variable S, combined with a high metafrenic acid level in the urine.

It can be concluded that the HRV variables described make it possible to differentiate between two sets of groups: firstly, to distinguish the high anxiety group from the low anxiety group, i.e. patients from staff; second, the stress reactor group from the non-stress reactor group, i.e. acute patients and neurotic staff, from chronic patients and stable staff.

On the basis of these results, we can only conclude that HR and HRV measurements can be a valuable new tool in psychiatry. First of all, HR and HRV is apparently relevant to the question 'how anxious is a person?' As this is often the main point in deciding whether to admit a person to a psychiatric hospital or not, and whether to indicate an intensive treatment or not, the HR and HRV measurements can be used to support these decisions one way or the other. Once a low S score has been found or a high HR or N, it is useful to continue taking HRV measurements on a weekly basis to see whether the variable S tends to increase, maybe indicating an improvement in the patient's condition. As there is 'normally' no difference in the HR and HRV scores made in repeated measurements, a change in HR and/or HRV score means, in our opinion, a change in 'mental state' or 'anxiety state'.

Compared with other measurement techniques, like questionnaires, observation scales, and the like, or EEG, EMG, etc., our technique has certain advantages. In the first place, the registration time is only 60 min. Second, the results are expressed numerically instead of verbally and they are immediately available because our special-purpose computer operates in real time. Third, the method can be repeated indefinitely. Fourth, for the HR and HRV scores active co-operation of the patient is unnecessary, which is a great advantage in psychiatry.

However, the method has its limitations since only one-third of the patients show 'abnormal' results i.e. below the 10 per cent value of the cumulative, adjusted frequency dispersion for the members of staff population. For these patients the method can give a useful indication of anxiety, whereas for the other 70 per cent of the patients it is of no special value.

Acknowledgements

This study was subsidized by the Organization for Health Research TNO. The author wishes to express his gratitude to Prof. Dr J. Bastiaans, Dr J. W. H. Kalsbeek, Dr P. F. Werre, Dr R. Jansen and Mr D. F. Sumter for their assistance in the research, and to Prof. Dr P. Visser for his constructive comments on the manuscript.

References

ACKER, C. W. (1964). An investigation of the variability in repeated psychophysiological measurements in tranquillized mental patients. *Psychophysiol.* **1** (2), 119–26.

BERGER, L. A. (1964). A comparison of the physiological functioning of normal and psychiatric patients. *Psycholog. Rep.* **15,** 183–7.

CROOKS, R. C. and McNULTY, J. A. (1966). Autonomic response specificity in normal and schizophrenic subjects. *Can. J. Psychol.* **20,** 280–95.

ETTEMA, J. H. (1967). Arbeidsfysiologische aspecten van mentale belasting [Work physiology aspects of mental load]. Van Gorkum, Assen.

FENZ, W. D. and VELNER, J. (1970). Physiological concomitants of behavioural indexes in schizophrenia. *J. abnorm. Psychol.* **76** (1), 27–35.

FLEKKÖY, K. and ASHUP, C. (1969). Psychophysiological responses of psychiatric patients related to social and other background factors. *Acta Nervosa*, Suppl. 11 (1), 36–41.

FRIEDMAN, H. P. and RUBIN, J. (1967). On some invariant criteria for grouping data. *Amer. stat. Assoc. J.* **62,** 1159–78.

KALSBEEK, J. W. H. (1967). Mentale belasting [Mental load]. Van Gorkum, Assen.

KELLY, D. H. and WALTER, C. J. (1968). The relationship between clinical diagnoses and anxiety, assessed by forearms bloodflow and other measurements. *Br. J. Psychiat.* **114** (510), 611–26.

——, BROWN, C. C., and SCHAFFER, J. W. (1970). A comparison of physiological and psychological measurements on anxious patients and normal subjects. *Psychophysiol.* **64,** 429–41.

LADER, M. H. and MATTHEUS, J. (1970). Physiological changes during spontaneous panic attacks. *J. psychosom. Res.* **14,** 377–82.

LEDER, S. (1966) Ueber den Verlauf von einigen physiologischen Reaktionen bei neurosen. [Physiological reactions in neurosis.] *Abh. Dt Akad. Wiss.* **2,** 313–23.

MILLER, W. H. and BERNAL, M. E. (1971). Measurements of the cardiac response in schizophrenic and normal children. *Psychophysiol.* 533–7.

MULDER, G. and MULDER, W. R. E. H. (1972). Heart rate variability in a binary choice relation task: an evaluation of some scoring methods. *Acta Psycholog.* **36,** 239–51.

OFFERHAUS, R. E. (1977a). Heart rate variability in a mental task situation. St. Bavò Research Report, St. Bavo Clinic, Noordwijkerhout.

—— (1977b). Heart rate variability and psychiatry. St. Bavo Research Report, St. Bavo Clinic, Noordwijkerhout.

PORGES, S. W. (1972). Heart rate variability and deceleration as indexes of reaction time. *J. exp. Psychol.* **92,** 103–10.

—— (1976). Peripheral and neurochemical parallels of psychopathology; A psychophysiological model relating autonomic imbalance to hyperactivity, psychopathy and autism. In *Advances in child development and behaviour* (ed. H. W. Reese). Academic Press, New York and London.

—— and RASKIN, D. C. (1969). Respiratory and heart rate components of attention. *J. exp. Psychol.* **81,** 497–503.

SHERMAN, M. (1945) Quantification of psychophysiological measures. *Psychosom. Med.* **7,** 215–19.

VARNI, J. G., CLARK, R. E., and GIDDON, D. B. (1971). Analysis of cyclic heart rate variability. *Psychophysiol.* **8,** 406–13.

WALTER, F. G. and PORGES, S. W. (1976). Heart Rate and respiratory responses as a function of task difficulty: the use of discriminant analysis in the selection of pscyhologically sensitive physiological responses. *Psychophysiol.* **13,** 563–71.

WIERSMA, E. D. (1913). Der Einfluss von Bewustseinszuständen auf den Puls und auf die Atmung [The influence of the state of consciousness on heart rate and respiration]. *Psych. en Neurol. Bladen.*

Concluding remarks

THE phenomenon of heart-rate variability (HRV) and its analysis has attracted the attention of workers in both pure and applied research and the contributions included here have reflected this. The material, however, is not intended to be complete and definitive. There are, for example, no contributions on respiratory sinus arrhythmia or on the relation between the results presented and physiological models of the circulation. Nevertheless, current research interests are well represented and certain general points drawn form this book warrant recapitulation.

The electrocardiogram (ECG) is a readily available source of physiological information. But the problem of reliable and accurate R-wave detection, as well as avoiding different types of artefacts, may still need attention (Byford). Moreover, the method for extracting significant information from the R-wave event series must be an explicit choice based upon a particular hypothesis of the underlying process (Sayers, Rompelman). A number of methods have been proposed for deriving HRV from the ECG. However, it is important to realize that the more sophisticated the analysis methods become, the more additional, uncertain factors are introduced. Such factors include the introduction of additional noise and uncertainty about confidence limits, e.g. the confidence limits of the power spectrum (Byford, Sayers).

The relation between the results of detailed analysis of R-wave event series and the proposed simplified models, such as the IPFM (Hyndman, Rompelman) and non-linear oscillatory control systems (Kitney, Rompelman) on the one hand and the physiology (McDonald, Noble, Sleight) on the other, is sometimes indicated (Kitney, Sayers); but it certainly needs much more elaboration.

It is interesting to note that in practical applications of HRV analysis the most commonly used statistical parameters are global, involving measuring the mean, the variance, etc. The problem with such measures is that they give the same result no matter what the order of the RR

239

intervals; where this can be confirmed by noting that randomizing the RR intervals results in large changes in the autocorrelation function or spectra of the signal (Sayers) and also in the pattern. It is important, therefore, to use techniques which employ the sequential properties of the signal, such as in the use of power in spectral bands as a set of HRV parameters (Hyndman). Other ways of parametrizing the HRV spectrum deserve further investigation. At present there is still some way to go before a full quantitative description of the physiology can be achieved. This process is likely to reveal other signal parameters which might prove more useful in fields such as psychiatry (Offerhaus) and mental-load investigations (Roscoe).

The application of HRV analysis in three areas of research: ergonomic studies, physiology, and in scoring procedures for psychology etc, covered by Luczak, Philipp, and Rohmert, shows another interesting aspect of the study of heart-rate variability. Many factors influence heart-rate, and some basic knowledge of the underlying generating processes, even if hypothetical, is essential when applying HRV analysis in any practical situation.

R.I.K.
O.R.

Index

accelerator nerve, *see* sympathetic control of heart rate
acetylcholine 18, 20
acidosis 8
action potential 4, 13
  frequency and temperature 17
  latency and single channel noise 15–17
adaption model 152
adrenaline 18, 19, 155, 158, 163, 164, 167, 213
afferent/efferent interface 202
afferent neural connection 202
age 5
air traffic controllers 214
aliasing 41–2
amplitude spectra 84
Amsterdam biographical questionnaire (ABQ) 236
annual variations 123
anxiety state 237
arousal 126, 143, 152, 154, 158, 164, 166, 167, 183, 232
ARQ measure 134, 144, 147, 163–7
arterial blood pressure 134, 140, 219
  control of by variations in heart rate 108
  essential hypertension 111
  long-term control of 111
  mean pressure 107
atrial mechanoreceptors 8, 9
atrio-ventricular node 3
autorhythmic effects 128, 131, 140
autocorrelation 121
automaticity of myocardial cells 3
autonomic activity 156, 197, 229
autonomic control of pacemaker 192
autonomic nervous system, reciprocity of 6, 7
autonomic regulatory processes 191
averaging process 119

Bainbridge reflex 8

bang-bang element 92, 95
baroreceptor control 202, 203, 207
baroreceptors 8, 167
  effect of denervation 111
  factors determining impulse frequency 110
  impulse frequency of 109
  linearity of response 110
  and long-term control of arterial blood pressure 111
  threshold 110
baroreflex
  gain 108, 211, 214
  and heart rate 107, 110
  and peripheral resistance 110
  testing of 110
behavioural activities 154
beta activity 155, 156, 163–6
Bezold–Jariseh reflex 8
binary choice 232
  capacity 235, 236
  generator 148, 228
  task 134, 140, 145, 168, 225, 226, 232
biochemical analyses 228
biochemical inhibitory mechanisms 215
blood pressure 6, 66, 67, 82, 124, 127, 132–4, 142, 191, 215–16
  elevated 215
  long-term control of 215
  mean arterial 32, 41
  spectrum 198
  spontaneous oscillations of 198
blood volume 216
bradycardia 8
brainstem 140, 156
Brown–Trigg approach 38–40, 55
bundle of His 3

cardiac cells, membrane properties 16–17
cardiac event 195, 198, 208
cardiac glycosides 20–2

cardiorespiratory influences 124–6, 138, 142, 154, 164, 167
cardiovascular reflexes 3, 7–9
cardiovascular regulatory processes 101, 191
carotid sinus 109, 138
  deterioration with age 111
carotid sinus nerve 7
carrier (free-running) frequency 193–4
catecholamines 126, 155, 156, 159, 163, 235
  concentration of 215
catheterization 191
central nervous influences 154, 156, 163, 164, 166
cerebellum 140
cerebral cortex 142
cerebrovisceral regulation disease 214
chemoreceptors 8
Chirp-Z transform 44
clonidine 110–11
cluster cell 192
cluster components 197
coefficient of variation 31, 42, 43, 56
cognitive task 208, 213
coherence function 70
coherent average 37, 53, 54, 55; see also ensemble average
coherent averaging 69, 71
complex demodulation 43, 52, 71–4, 84
components 32, 46, 48, 51, 52, 56
computer simulation 203
consciousness 225
control 81, 214
  humoral 154, 167
  neural 156
  non-linear 66, 67
  oscillating 65
control theory 90, 126
  model of 90
convolution 44
correlation 85, 117
  auto- 29, 30, 33, 36, 37
  coefficient 33, 54
  cross 42, 84
  event auto- 31
  non-circular 42
  serial 29, 30, 34, 35, 37
correlation function
  auto- 69–71
  cross 69–71
cortex 142
cortical influences 154

covariance 33
crossing point 101
cuff pressure 216, 218
cyclic factors 121

decaying oscillation 95
degrees of freedom 29, 33, 34, 35, 36, 38, 42, 43, 54, 121
  per point 29, 33, 34, 35, 36
delays, frequency dependent 120
depolarization of cardiac cells 4, 13, 14
  rate of 15, 16, 18
depressor nerve, see vagus nerve
describing function 67, 96, 100
  technique 95
diastole 4
diastolic pressure 107
Dirac pulse 37, 40
disturbance signal 198
  HF 199
diurnal variations 124
dual input describing function (DIDF) 96, 100, 101

ECG 59, 61, 65, 143, 159, 191
EEG 154–6, 159, 164–7
efferent activity, CVS sympathetic 202, 203
ego strength 235
electromyographic influences 155
emotional influences 149, 152, 154, 158, 163, 164, 167, 169
endocrine influences 156
ensemble 31, 34, 35, 36, 42, 53, 54, 55, average 37, 38
entrainment 68, 81, 83, 86, 89, 90, 95, 96, 101–4, 123, 143, 199, 201, 206, 207, 211
ergonomic analysis 123, 126
ergonomic physiology 60
error 33, 38, 42, 51
  forecasting 38
  signal 38
  smoothed rectified 38
essential hypertension, aetiology of 191
event detection 209
event process analysis 59, 60
event spectrum 198
exercise 3, 5, 9
  and baroreflex 107, 110
external stimulus 96, 98, 99, 100, 101, 199
extra systoles 21

factor analysis 229
feature analysis 55, 56
fiducial point 118
filter 39, 45
  band-selective 43, 44, 45, 46, 47, 48,
    49, 56
  homomorphic 71, 75
  linear 69, 71
  low-pass 44, 47, 52
  matched 69, 71
  moving average 45
  trend 55
  zero-phase-shift 44
Fourier transform 44, 72, 121
  fast Fourier transform (FFT) 44
  inverse 50
frequency 42, 43, 51, 52
  domain 42, 46, 69
  heart 225
  oscillation 100
fundamental component 99

gain of baroreflex 108
  and clonidine 110–11
  and environmental factors 111
  and exercise 110
  and hypertension 110
Gaussian 28, 37, 42, 43, 54, 56
gravitational stress 118

harmonic 31, 37, 45, 47, 53
homeostasis 202
  blood pressure 212
hormone increases 213
humoral control 154, 167
hypercapnia 8
hypothalamus 142, 156
hypoxia 8

impulse train 193, 194
information processing 124, 152–5, 158,
  163
  handling task 168
  load 152
input information rate 149, 156
instability 104
instantaneous rate 118
integral pulse frequency modulation
  (IPFM) 103, 198, 205
intelligence tests 235
interval 28–32, 35, 37–45, 50–3, 55, 57
  mean 35, 39, 45–6, 56
  inter-beat 27, 28, 30, 32, 39, 43

spectrum 45, 55
interval function 61
interval reflex model 205
interval tachogram 82
intrathoracic pressure 132, 207
intravascular pressure 218
invasive measurements 191
inward background current 15

Kolmogorov–Smirnov test 51

length bias 32
linear characteristics 92, 95, 198
locus 92
low frequency component 97
low frequency disturbance 198
low pass filter 118
low pass filtered event series (LPFES) 61,
  83, 197
  spectrum of 84, 85, 86, 90
lymbic system 154

mass 5
medication, anti-psychotic 235
medulla 156
  vasomotor centres 3, 7
membrane potential
  intracellular recording of 4
  resting potential 4, 192
mental capacity 153
mental load 125, 143, 147–9, 153, 155,
  168, 169, 183, 185, 214, 225
mental state 237
mental strain 148, 168, 169
mental task 145, 232
mental work 124, 167
metabolic 168
metafrenic acid 236
metastable entrainment 83, 87, 88, 89, 90,
  103
metastability 86, 90, 104
Minnesota multiphasic personality inventory
  (MMPI) scales 235, 236
mode
  on 202
  off 202
modulation frequency 194
moments, of distribution 33
motor action 145, 151
movement observations 228
multiple choice task 148, 155

natural oscillation 99–101
  frequency 102–4

negative exponential 43, 45
negative feedback 92
negative phase 98
neural cardiovascular system 59
neural control 156
neurotic influences 214, 236
non-linear HRV 50, 51, 82
non-linear oscillatory systems 81
non-linear switch 92, 95
non-linear system 103–4, 199, 202
non-linearity 95–101, 204
non-stationarity 31, 34, 35, 38, 39, 55, 56, 120
non-stress reactor group 236
noradrenaline 18, 110, 155
Nyquist criterion 200
Nyquist locus 93, 94, 102
Nyquist plane 93, 95
Nyquist plot 92, 201
Nyquist rate 42

open-loop transfer function 93
oscillations 66, 68, 76, 81, 90, 168
  frequency 94, 105
  non-stationary 68, 74
  self-sustained 96
  spontaneous 3, 199–202, 207
output waveform 97, 99

pacemaker frequency 191
pacemaker potential 13–14
  and acetylcholine 20
  and catecholamines 18–19
  ionic currents involved 14–15
  and temperature 17
parasympathetic influences 62, 154, 156
pattern 27, 28, 31, 34, 35, 37, 39, 47, 50, 52, 53, 54, 55
  analysis 32, 52
period, oscillation of the 94
periodicity 31, 42, 52, 54
peripheral smooth muscle 105
peripheral vascular bed 92, 215
peripheral vascular resistance 93, 132–3, 205
peripheral vasoconstriction 7, 8, 111
peripheral vasodilation 110
perspective plotting 86, 88
phase 35, 36, 37, 44, 46
  spectrum 34, 35, 43, 46, 48, 49, 50, 56
phasic arousal 154, 156, 167–9
phenylephrine 110
photoplethysmogram 82, 216, 218

physical work load 138
physiological state 117
pilot workload 178, 179, 182, 189
point event 27, 31, 40, 41
  sequence 41
positive phase 98
potassium current 14, 18, 19
  Q_{10} of 17
power 37, 42, 43, 45, 86
  a.c. 42, 51
  distribution 89
  relative 211
  signal 29, 33, 34, 56
  spectrum 34, 35, 38, 42, 50, 70, 82, 83, 84, 196, 197
  spontaneous 86
  total 86, 210
  variability 37, 56
PP-interval 61
pressoreceptors 132
pressure vasomotor 44, 46, 48, 52
  oscillations 44, 50
PR-interval 61
probability 54
  density function 37
psychiatry 225, 226
psychic apparatus 225
psychic state 225, 229
psychic stress 153, 156
psychological state 117
psychological stress 191
psychological testing 228, 235
psychopharmacological medication 235
psychophysical influences 167
psychosocial environment 191
psychotic influences 235
pulse amplitude 225
pulse interval 107
pulse pressure 107, 110
pure-time delay 92, 93, 94, 96, 104
Purkinje cells 3
Purkinje fibres 17, 18
P-wave 59

quenched oscillation 100, 102

radio telemetry 159
reaction time factor (RTF) 155–6
refractory period 192, 193, 210
repolarization of cardiac cells 4
respiration 124, 127, 128, 132, 159, 164, 165, 167, 198, 226
respiratory arrhythmia 66, 127, 134, 225

respiratory control systems 82
respiratory cycle 118, 126, 140
respiratory influences 45, 46, 52, 56
respiratory sinus arrhythmia 8
rest-mental task analyses 226
reticular influences 154
rhythms 143
RR interval 59–61, 143
  spectrum 82
  waveform 82, 83
running coherence 84
running correlation average 84
running phase spectrum 90
running power 84
running spectra 84
R-wave 59, 63
  spike train 191
sample, statistical 29, 41, 56
  sampling effects 29, 31
schizophrenia 235
seasonal variations 124
sequence 29, 31, 39, 41, 45
  interval 32, 38, 39, 46, 48, 56
sequence point event 41
sequence randomized 29
signal analysis 68
single-input describing function 99, 101
sino-artrial node 3, 5, 13, 15, 17, 22, 41
  artery 5
  entrainment of discharge rate 5
sinus arrhythmia 39, 46, 125, 179, 183,
  191
  as an indicator of work load 183–5
sinus (SA) node 59, 60, 62, 133
sleep 124, 154
smooth muscle 105, 202, 205
socio-economic stressors 191
sodium/calcium current 15, 19, 20
sodium current 15
sodium–potassium exchange pump 19, 20
somatic influences 143, 156
spectral analysis 65, 66, 123, 127, 155
spectral density 31, 35, 51
spectral running 69
spectral window 194, 195
spectrum 29, 33, 37, 41, 48, 51, 55,
  amplitude 34, 35, 36, 37, 43, 46, 48, 49,
    50
  interval 32, 56
  phase 34, 35, 43, 46, 48, 49, 50, 56
  power 34, 35, 38, 42, 50
sphygmamometer cuff 218
spinal cord 140

stable limit cycle 101
stable oscillation 95, 100
stable thermal component 86
standard deviation 32, 34, 42, 43, 53, 54,
  56
standard error 29, 33, 34, 35, 56
startle reactions 229
stationarity 32, 39, 43, 55
stimulus frequency 86, 104
strain 123, 125, 159, 168, 169
stress 125, 155, 158, 167
stress-induced hypertension 213
stressor influences 123, 158, 163, 167
stress reactor group 236
stretch receptors 127
sustained oscillation 95, 100
switch element (threshold device) 95, 98,
  101, 200, 202
sympathetic influences 62, 133, 142, 143,
  156
sympathetic control of heart rate 18, 108–
  9
sympathetic system 6, 8
  ionotropic effects 8
systems analysis 125
systolic pressure 107

tachogram 60, 63, 226, 228
tachycardia 7, 8
task 143, 152, 155, 158, 159, 168, 169,
  213
Tauber waves 118
test–retest analyses 226, 229
thermal component 103
thermal entrainment 82
thermal influences 45, 51, 56, 82, 168
thermal regulation 3, 9
thermal stimuli 82, 87, 90
thermoregulation 81
thermoregulatory mechanism 124
thermoregulatory system 66, 67
theta activity 155, 156, 163–7
threshold potential 4
threshold value 193
time domain 41
tonic arousal 154, 158, 164–7, 169
tracking signal 38, 39, 40
transient inward current 15
transition phenomenon 103
trend 38, 39, 55
  detection 39
  linear 40, 42
  test 38

unstable amplitude 86
unstable entrainment 84, 90, 91, 102, 103
unstable oscillations 84, 95
unsystematic influences 229
urinary biochemical component 236
urine 158, 159

vagus nerve 6, 8, 13, 108–9
vascular nerves 133
vascular muscles 133
vasomotor activity 81
vasomotor centre 132, 133

vasomotor system 132
vasomotor tone 138
vagal influences 62, 133, 142, 143
venomotor tone 205
ventricular contractility, left 205
ventricular mechanoreceptors 8
voltage-clamp technique 13, 20

wakefulness 154
waveform 84
weighting function 194, 195
work load 123, 125, 134, 142, 155, 168
wrap-around effects 44, 46, 48, 56